Pocket Guide to Colorectal Cancer

Jones and Bartlett Series in Oncology

Pocket Guide to Colorectal Cancer

Deborah T. Berg, RN, BSN
Oncology Consultant
Derry, New Hampshire

JONES AND BARTLETT PUBLISHERS
Sudbury, Massachusetts
BOSTON   TORONTO   LONDON   SINGAPORE

World Headquarters

Jones and Bartlett Publishers	Jones and Bartlett Publishers Canada	Jones and Bartlett Publishers International
40 Tall Pine Drive	2406 Nikanna Road	Barb House, Barb Mews
Sudbury, MA 01776	Mississauga,	London W6 7PA
978-443-5000	ON L5C 2W6	UK
info@jbpub.com	CANADA	
www.jbpub.com		

Library of Congress Cataloging-in-Publication Data

Berg, Deborah T.
    Pocket guide to colorectal cancer / Deborah T. Berg.
      p. cm
    Includes bibliographical references and index.
    ISBN: 0-7637-0172-6
    1. Colon (Anatomy)–Cancer–Nursing–Handbooks, manuals, etc. 2. Rectum–Cancer–Nursing–Handbooks, manuals, etc. I. Title.
    [DNLM: 1. Colorectal Neoplasms–Handbooks. WI 39 B493p 2002]
    RC280.C6 B47 2002
    616.99'4347–dc21

                             2002034163

Acquisitions Editor: Penny M. Glynn
Production Manager: Amy Rose
Associate Production Editor: Karen C. Ferreira
Associate Editor: Karen Zuck
Production Assistant: Jenny McIsaac
Senior Marketing Manager: Alisha Weisman
Marketing Associate: Joy Stark-Vancs
Manufacturing and Inventory Coordinator: Amy Bacus
Cover Design: Philip Regan
Interior Design: Modern Graphics
Composition: Northeast Compositors
Printing and Binding: United Graphics
Cover Printing: United Graphics

Printed in the United States of America
06 05 04 03 02   10 9 8 7 6 5 4 3 2 1

Dedication

"To the courage and dedication of our patients, whose today is filled with anxiety, and whose tomorrow is unpredictable."

Maimonides (12th century philosopher/physician)

May we as nurses never forget the difference our knowledge and skills can make to patients and their families.

With love and appreciation to my husband, Ed, and my daughters, Megan and Lauren. Your love and support are extraordinary.

Contents

The authors, editor, and publisher have made every effort to provide accurate information.

However, they are not responsible for errors, omissions, or for any outcomes related to the use of the contents of this book and take no responsibility for the use of the products described. Drugs and medical devices are discussed that may have limited availability controlled by the Food and Drug Administration (FDA) for use only in a research study or clinical trial. The drug information presented has been derived from reference sources, recently published data, and pharmaceutical tests. Research, clinical practice, and government regulations often change the accepted standard in this field. When consideration is being given to use of any drug in the clinical setting, the health care provider or reader is responsible for determining FDA status of the drug, reading the package insert, and prescribing information for the most up-to-date recommendations on dose, precautions, and contraindications and determining the appropriate usage of the product. This is especially important in the case of drugs that are new or seldom used.

Preface

Welcome to the first edition of the *Pocket Guide for Colorectal Cancer*. The goal of this pocket guide is to provide an easy-to-use, practical reference for nurses who care for patients with colorectal cancer. To help nurses use this guide, the content is divided into five parts:

◆ The Basics About Colorectal Cancer: Epidemiology, Screening/Early Detection, and Prevention

◆ Disease Assessment

◆ Primary Cancer of the Colon and Rectum: Therapeutic Approaches and Nursing Care

◆ Treatment of Recurrent and Metastatic Colorectal Cancer

◆ Care of the Individual with Colorectal Cancer

This pocket guide reflects the updated content drawn from *Contemporary Issues in Colorectal Cancer: A Nursing Perspective*. Three appendices are also available with a resource section and information about toxicity descriptions. However, colorectal cancer is an area of dynamic, active investigation; therefore, care is undergoing rapid changes.

Colorectal cancer is preventable, detectable, and treatable when we are all correctly informed about the risk factors, prevention methods, screening recommendations, and treatment options. As nurses we must remember that no matter how our day is going, the patient surviving colorectal cancer is facing a serious, probably life-threatening illness. By being informed, taking time to listen, and providing the best physical and psychological care possible, we can make a great difference in the lives of patients and their families.

Acknowledgements

This resource book would not have been possible if not for the foresight of Jones and Bartlett Publishers. I would like to thank Penny Glynn for her support throughout the creation of the manuscript and Amy Rose, who was instrumental in its final development. It was your time, patience, attention to detail, and persistence that made this a book of which to be proud. The content provided by the contributors of *Contemporary Issues in Colorectal Cancer: A Nursing Perspective* was invaluable. I therefore wish to acknowledge the following nurses and physicians for their willingness to share their expertise:

Kathy Christiansen, RN, BSN, OCN
Mary Ellen Crane, RN, BSN, CETN

Denise A. DeLollo, RN, OCN

Tracy K. Gosselin, RN, MSN, AOCN

Joyce P. Griffin-Sobel, RN, PhD, AOCN, CS

Cathering M. Hogan, MN, RN, CS, AOCN

Cynthia R. King, PhD, NP, MSN, RN, FAAN

Yvonne Lassere, RN, OCN, CCRP

Neal Meropol, MD

Marilyn Mulay, RN, MS, OCN

Delores A. Saddler, RN, MSN, CGRN

Margot R. Sweed, RN, CRNP, CNSN

Anne R. Waldman, MSN, RN, C, AOCN

Finally, but certainly not least, thanks to my family, Larry and Betty Anderson, Anna and Russell Peter Berg. Thanks to my husband Ed and daughters Megan and Lauren for encouraging me, guiding me, and understanding that such ventures are time consuming.

PART I

The Basics About Colorectal Cancer: Epidemiology, Screening/Early Detection, and Prevention

1

Epidemiology Trends: Incidence and Survival

Introduction

"Colorectal" refers to the colon and rectum, which together make up the large intestine, also known as the large bowel. Colorectal cancer (CRC) is cancer of the colon or rectum. Cancer of the colon and rectum is a major health problem worldwide, and in the United States, it is one of the most prevalent malignancies, utilizing a significant proportion of our healthcare dollars. Moreover, there is no group for which these tumors are **not** a major health problem.

Trends in Incidence

❖ Third most common malignancy (after prostate and lung cancer in men and after breast and lung cancer in women)[1]

❖ Lifetime risk approximately 6%[1]

❖ Estimated 148,300 new cases in 2002[1]

  ❖ 107,300 total new cases in the colon

   50,000 new cases in men

   57,300 new cases in women

  ❖ 41,000 total new cases in the rectum

   22,600 new cases in men

   18,400 new cases in women

❖ Incidence decreased between 1985 and 1995 at a rate of about 2% per year.[2]

  ❖ Trend observed in both men and women of all racial and ethnic groups (data insufficient for American Indian women)[3]

  ❖ Declining incidence attributed to increased public and professional awareness of CRC, assimilation of recommended dietary habits, and screening/removal of polyps

❖ Incidence increased between 1995 and 1998 at a rate of approximately 0.5%.[2]

  ❖ Increasing incidence attributed to increases in early detection

  ❖ Anticipate continued increase in incidence as U.S. population ages unless prevention and screening are improved

❖ Tumors of the proximal colon are becoming more common.[4]

❖ Geography

  ❖ Incidence higher in industrialized regions

1. World areas with highest incidence: Eastern and Western Europe, Scandinavian countries, New Zealand, Australia, Canada, and the United States[1]

❖ In the United States, the highest incidence is noted in:

1. States or areas with current or previous intense industrialization
2. The east compared with the west and the north compared with the south[5]
3. Rural areas compared with urban area[5]

❖ There is no link between incidence and occupational exposure.[5]

❖ Table 1-1 shows the states within the United States with the highest and lowest incidence.

TABLE 1-1
States within the United States with the Highest and Lowest Incidence of Colorectal Cancer: Top 10 List[1]

State	Rate per 100,000	State	Rate per 100,000
California	12, 900	New Hampshire	700
Florida	10,400	Idaho	600
New York	10,400	South Dakota	500
Texas	9,500	Hawaii	500
Pennsylvania	8,700	Montana	500
Ohio	7,200	Delaware	400
Illinois	6,800	North Dakota	400
Michigan	5,300	Vermont	400
New Jersey	4,900	Wyoming	300
Massachusetts	3,800	Alaska	200

Trends in Survival and Mortality

❖ Second leading cause of cancer-related deaths after lung cancer

❖ Mortality rates differ by region.

❖ Estimated 56,600 deaths in 2002[1]

  ❖ 48,100 deaths due to colon cancer[1]

   23,100 deaths in men

   25,000 deaths in women

  ❖ 8,500 deaths due to rectal cancer[1]

   4,700 deaths in men

   3,800 deaths in women

❖ Mortality decreased between 1990 and 1996 at a rate of 1.7% per year.[3]

❖ Factors relating to decreased mortality[6]

  ❖ Better surgical techniques: wider margins, modern anesthetics, and improved supportive care

  ❖ Better pathologic and preoperative staging

  ❖ Use of adjuvant systemic chemotherapy for colon cancers and chemoradiotherapy for rectal cancers

❖ Access to health insurance may influence patient outcomes.[7]

  ❖ Uninsured patients have a mortality rate 64% higher than those insured.

  ❖ Medicaid patients fare better than the uninsured; mortality rate is 36% higher than patients with private insurance.

TABLE 1–2
Five-Year Survival by Stage[1]

Stage	5-Year Survival
Localized disease	90%
Regional disease	65%
Metastatic disease	8%

* Patients with health maintenance organizations have a mortality rate 22% higher than fee-for-service private insurance plans.[7]

* The percentage of people alive at 5 years is improving and is greatly influenced by the stage of disease at the time of diagnosis.

* Survival decreases with advanced stage of disease at diagnosis.

* Table 1-2 shows 5-year survival by stage.

Gender, Racial, and Ethnic Differences in Incidence and Mortality

* Gender
  * Incidence nearly equal in men and women
    1. Accounts for 11% and 12% of all new cancer cases in American men and women respectively[1]
    2. Cumulative lifetime risk is nearly equal: men 1 in 17 and women 1 in 18[1]
    3. Between 1985 and 1995, decrease in incidence is slightly greater in men rather than in women.[2]

❖ Tumor location differs slightly by gender.[6]
  1. Women more frequently diagnosed with colon tumors
  2. Men more commonly diagnosed with rectal tumors
❖ Mortality nearly equal between men and women
  1. Accounts for 10% and 11% of cancer-related deaths in American men and women, respectively[1]
  2. Is the third leading cause of cancer-related mortality, respectively (after lung and prostate cancer in men and lung and breast cancer in women)[1]

❖ Race and ethnicity
  ❖ Incidence and mortality rates vary by race and ethnicity.
  ❖ Between 1985 and 1995, decrease in incidence and mortality noted.
    1. Decline in incidence is considerably greater in whites than in African Americans.[2]
    2. Decline in mortality is similar between men and women, but greater in whites than in African Americans.[2]
    3. African Americans, both men and women, have the highest incidence and mortality of all racial or ethnic groups.
  ❖ Table 1-3 shows the incidence and mortality rates by race and ethnicity.

❖ Stage of disease at diagnosis differs slightly by race.

    1. All ethnic groups present with similar stages of disease, except African Americans.[8]

TABLE 1-3
Incidence and Mortality Rates by Race and Ethnicity, United States:* 1990–1997[1]

Racial/Ethnic Group	Incidence	Mortality
White		
(Total)	42.9	16.8
Men	51.4	20.6
Women	36.3	13.9
African American		
(Total)	50.1	22.8
Men	57.7	27.3
Women	44.7	19.6
Asian/Pacific Islander		
(Total)	38.2	10.7
Men	47.3	12.9
Women	31.0	8.9
American Indian/Alaska Native		
(Total)	28.6	10.3
Men	33.5	11.9
Women	24.6	8.9
Hispanic		
(Total)	28.4	10.2
Men	35.2	13.0
Women	23.2	8.0

*Rates are per 100,000

2. African Americans present more often with metastatic disease.[1]

3. Reasons are unclear for this disparity, but the following are possible factors for difference in stage at presentation:

   a. Poverty and poor access to medical care are often cited, but do not answer why this is a factor for only *one* minority population.

   b. Genetic makeup, tumor pathology, or another undiscovered factor may be involved.

❖ Possible factors associated with higher mortality in different race and ethnic groups: tumor pathology, comorbid conditions and potential differences in treatment

References

1. Jemal A, Thomas A, Murray T, and Thun M. "Cancer Statistics, 2002." *CA Cancer J Clin.* 2002; 52(1): 23–47.

2. Ries LA, Eisner MP, Kosary CL, *et al.* (ed). *SEER Cancer Statistics Review, 1973–1998.* Bethesda, MD: National Cancer Institute, 2001.

3. Greenlee RT, Murray T, Bolden S, *et al.* "Cancer Statistics, 2000." *CA Cancer J Clin.* 2000; 50(1): 7–33.

4. DeVita V, Hellman S, and Rosenberg S. *Cancer: Principles and Practices of Oncology,* 6th ed. Philadelphia, PA: Lippincott-Raven, 2001.

5. Goldberg RM. "Gastrointestinal Tract Cancers." In Casciato DA, and Lowitz BB, eds. *Manual of Clinical*

Oncology, 4th ed. Philadelphia, PA: Lippincott Williams & Wilkins, 2000: 182–194.

6. Ellenhorn JDI, Coia LR, Alberts SR, and Hoff PM. "Colorectal and Anal Cancers." In Pazdur R, Coia LR, Hoskins HJ, and Wagman LD, eds. *Cancer Management: A Multidisciplinary Approach*, 6th ed. Melville, NY: PRR, Inc, 2002: 295–318.

7. Reuters News. "Colorectal Cancer Mortality Higher Among Blacks and the Uninsured." Available at http://oncology.medscape.com/reuters/prof/2000/11/11 .06/20001103epid002.html. Accessed November 15, 2000.

8. Jessup JM, McGinnis LS, Steele GD, *et al.* "The National Cancer Data Base Report on Colon Cancer." *Cancer.* 1996; 78: 918–926.

2

Risk Factors: The Role of Hereditary, Environmental, and Dietary Factors

Introduction

The specific cause of colon and rectum cancer (CRC) is unknown. There are several intrarelated factors under investigation. Environmental, nutritional, inherited factors, and preexisting diseases are all associated with this cancer. Risk factors—inherited and non-inherited—pose a major concern and are a source of considerable confusion. While approximately 75% of all cancers of the colon or rectum occur sporadically, about 25% are associated with familial or inherited factors.

Major Risk Factors

❖ A risk factor is a trait or characteristic that has been confirmed scientifically to be associated with an increased incidence of a certain disease.

After risk factors are identified, the appropriate prevention and detection methods are selected.

❖ Main risk factors are increasing age, preexisting adenomatous polyps or adenomas, family history, genetic predisposition, preexisting disease of the bowel, and environmental factors.[1]

Increasing Age

❖ CRC is considered a disease of the elderly.

❖ CRC is rare before the age of 30.[2]

❖ Incidence increases with age.[2]

  ❖ Risk is 1 in 1,508 in men and 1 in 1,719 in women before the age of 39.
  ❖ Risk is 1 in 115 in men and 1 in 145 in women between the ages of 40 and 59.
  ❖ Risk is 1 in 25 in men and 1 in 33 in women between the ages of 60 and 79.
  ❖ Risk doubles with each decade after the age of 50.
  ❖ More than 90% of new diagnoses occur after the age of 50 years.
  ❖ Risk declines after the 8th or 9th decade.

❖ The median age at diagnosis is 67 years.[1]

❖ Inverse relationship between age and stage of disease at diagnosis without impact on survival[3]

  ❖ Patients under the age of 50 present with more advanced-stage disease, while those over the age of 80 years present with early-stage disease.

1. Despite more advanced disease, younger patients have a 14% to 24% improvement in survival compared with the older adult.
2. Patients 70–79 years of age had a 4% to 9% improvement in survival compared with the oldest patients, age > 80.[3]

❖ Possible factors for inverse relationship between age and stage at diagnosis while no real impact on survival
1. Comorbid conditions and postoperative complications
2. Possible disparity in adjuvant chemotherapy and radiotherapy, i.e., older patients may not be offered adjuvant therapy[4,5]

❖ Careful selection of patients for surgery and systemic chemotherapy, based on functional (performance) status, not on age, is key to the elderly patient receiving the same therapeutic benefit as younger patients.[4-7]

Adenomatous Polyps or Adenomas

❖ Polyps are the precursor lesions to cancers of the colon and rectum.

❖ Polyps become more common with age.[8]
  ❖ About 30% of people in their 50s produce polyps.
  ❖ About 50% of people in their 70s produce polyps.[8]
  ❖ People who produce polyps are more likely to develop CRC than people who do not produce polyps.[1]

❖ Histologically, there are two general types of polyps.[9]

  ❖ Nonneoplastic
    1. No malignant potential: hyperplastic, mucous retention, hamartomas (juvenile) lymphoid aggregates, and inflammatory polyps[9]

  ❖ Neoplastic
    1. Have malignant potential
    2. Adenomatous polyps account for 70% of polyps removed at endoscopic examination.[9]

❖ Adenomas are classified by their structure.

  ❖ Pedunculated (stalked or tubular) account for 75–85% of polyps.[9]
  ❖ Sessile (flat or villous) account for about 5%.[9]
  ❖ Tubulovillous, a combination of the two, account for about 10% to 25%.[9]

❖ Most polyps do not become cancerous, but a subset can under the influence of genetic events.

  ❖ Polyps are present for several years before they potentially evolve into cancer; as the polyp enlarges, an adenoma forms; it becomes more dysplastic, developing into a carcinoma in situ, then into an invasive cancer if not removed.
  ❖ There is a 5% chance that a polyp will become malignant.[1]

❖ Factors predictive of malignant transformation of a polyp

- Sessile and tubulovillous polyps are associated with a higher frequency of malignant transformation.[1]
- Polyps with high-grade dysplasia are more likely to become malignant.[9]
- Polyps that are severely dysplastic become malignant in approximately 3.5 years while those with mild atypia progress in about 11.5 years.[9]
- Individuals with multiple polyps have a five- to sevenfold increased risk of them becoming malignant.[9]
- Risk of malignant transformation increases with size of the polyp.[1]

  1. Polyps of less than 1 cm have about a 1% risk of becoming malignant.
  2. Polyps greater than 2 cm have about a 40% likelihood of becoming malignant.
  3. About 2.5% of polyps larger than 1 cm progress by 5 years; 8% by 10 years; and 24% by 20 years.[9]

- There is an opportunity for screening and early detection modalities. The first goal would be to screen individuals, remove polyps before they become malignant, thereby preventing CRC. The second goal is to detect CRC early, thereby decreasing mortality. Polypectomy and continued surveillance can reduce the incidence of CRC by about 90% compared with individuals not screened.[9]

Familial and Genetic Factors

❖ Cancers, including CRC, develop because cells change as a result of some genetic mischance, either present since birth (germline defects) or occurring later due to a mutation caused by a toxic exposure (somatic mutations).

❖ People with a personal history of cancer have an increased risk of developing another cancer.[1]

  ❖ People with previous CRC are at increased risk of developing a second CRC or a cancer in another location.

  ❖ Women with breast, endometrial, or ovarian cancers are at increased risk of developing CRC.

❖ People with a family history of CRC have an increased risk of developing CRC.[1]

  ❖ The risk increases two- to threefold for individuals with a family history involving a first-degree relative diagnosed with CRC. The risk is highest if the first-degree relative was diagnosed before the age of 60 and if there are multiple first-degree relatives or affected family members regardless of the age at diagnosis. The risk increases further in the presence of a genetic familial syndrome.[10,11]

  ❖ Table 2-1 outlines the association of family history on the risk of developing CRC.

  ❖ The familial-genetic link (or factor) may be a common exposure among family members, environmental consequences, or some combination of these.[9]

TABLE 2-1
Association of Family History on the Risk of Colorectal Cancer Development.[10,11]

Overall risk	6%
Negative family history of colorectal cancer	2%
Positive family history	
• first-degree relative with CRC	6%
• first-degree relative plus	
• two second-degree relatives with CRC	8%
• first-degree relative diagnosed < age 45	10%
• first-degree relatives with CRC	17%
Genetic syndromes	
• HNPCC (genetic carrier)	70%
• FAP (genetic carrier)	100%

Note: A first-degree relative is a parent, sibling, or child; a second-degree relative is an aunt, uncle, or cousin. CRC, colorectal cancer. HNPCC, hereditary nonpolyposis colon cancer; FAP, familial adenomatous polyposis.

❖ Specific genetic mutations have been detected in some cancer-prone families, accounting for 5% to 6% of all colorectal cancer[12]
❖ As yet undiscovered major genetic mutations and/or background genetic factors may also contribute to the development of CRC

Genetic Syndromes

❖ There are two main genetic syndromes
  ❖ Familial adenomatous polyposis (FAP)
  ❖ Hereditary nonpolyposis colorectal cancer (HNPCC)

❖ The characteristics of these syndromes differ, yet they share the polyp to adenoma to cancer sequence with each other and with sporadic CRC.

❖ There are other rare genetic syndromes.[1]

1. Gardner's syndrome, a variant of FAP, with the addition of extracolonic features
2. Turcot's syndrome, also a variant of FAP, is characterized by colon and brain tumors.
3. Peutz-Jeghers' and juvenile polyposis syndromes are not cancerous or precancerous conditions, but are associated with an increased risk of developing CRC.

❖ Familial adenomatous polyposis (FAP)

❖ Inherited autosomal dominant syndrome, risk of CRC 100%

❖ FAP accounts for 1% of the CRC incidence, which represents about 7,000 people.[12]

❖ Typical clinical scenario[1,12]

1. Polyps develop early, on average by the age of 25.

   a. Polyps are not usually present at birth.
   b. 50% of patients develop polyps by the age of 15.
   c. 95% of patients develop polyps by the age of 35.

2. There are hundreds to thousands of polyps, usually pedunculated, spread throughout the colon.
3. Symptoms usually develop by the age of 33.
4. FAP is diagnosed by the age of 36.

5. Colorectal cancer is diagnosed by the age of 42 (range 34–43 years).
6. Extracolonic characteristics include mandibular osteomas, upper gastrointestinal polyps, and congenital hypertrophy of the retinal pigment epithelium.

❖ The adenomatous polyposis coli (APC) gene predisposes people to FAP.

1. APC gene is found in about 80% of families with this syndrome.[13]
2. It is a tumor-suppressor gene.

❖ Genetic testing is recommended for families with known FAP, especially if the affected person has a positive APC test.[13]

1. If the affected relative is positive and the family member is negative, that family member is considered at average risk for development of CRC.[13]

❖ Screening recommendations for these high-risk families are outlined in Chapter 3, Table 3–3.[13]

❖ Standard management involves a total colectomy with construction of an ileal pouch–anal anastomosis.[13]

1. The nonsteriodal antiinflammatory agent, sulindac, and the cyclooxygenase-2 inhibitor, celecoxib, have demonstrated a benefit in terms of decreasing the size and number of polyps. Only celecoxib is FDA approved as an adjunct to standard management.[1]

❖ The genetic mutation APCI1307K is an alteration of the APC gene.

    ❖ Inherited mutation that does not directly lead to CRC, but rather makes the gene more susceptible to additional genetic changes that can result in CRC.[14]

        1. Confers a 10–20% increase risk in developing CRC[14]

    ❖ It is believed that 6% of people from Eastern Europe of Ashkenazi Jewish descent carry this mutation.[14]

        1. Genetic testing for any person of Ashkenazi heritage who either has a personal or a family history of CRC or polyps is recommended.

        2. Testing for this mutation is extremely accurate; a positive result is truly positive.[14]

        3. Parents who are positive for APCI1307K have a 50% chance of passing the mutation on to each offspring.[14]

    ❖ If the test is positive, routine screening with colonoscopy for CRC is recommended.[14]

    ❖ More research into this mutation and the afflicted population is needed.

❖ Hereditary Nonpolyposis Colon Cancer (HNPCC)

    ❖ Inherited autosomal dominant syndrome; it is more common than FAP, accounting for 5% of the CRC incidence or about 1 in every 500 people.[12]

    ❖ Clinically, HNPCC looks like sporadic CRC.

1. Polyps are scattered within the colon.[12]
2. Polyps progress through the carcinogenesis sequence but at an accelerated pace compared with sporadic cancers.[13]
3. Cancers commonly arise in the right colon.[12]
4. People with this syndrome tend to develop cancer at an early age; mean age 44 compared to 68 for general population.[9,12]
5. Is associated with cancers outside of the colon (extracolonic) tumors: primarily breast, endometrial, ovarian, kidney, stomach, biliary tract, brain, and small intestine.[12]
6. The prognosis is better than for those with sporadic cancer; HNPCC death rate is two thirds that of sporadic CRC over a 10-year period.[9]

❖ HNPCC is divided into two variants.

1. Lynch I is associated with CRC only.
2. Lynch II is associated with CRC and with extracolonic cancers.[9]

❖ Genetic changes in the mismatch repair (MMR) genes predispose for HNPCC.

1. Known MMR genes include hMSH1, hMLH1, hPMS1, hPMS2, hMSH3, and hMSH6.[1]
2. Genetic testing may be helpful, but since only a few MMR genes have been identified, some families may still have HNPCC but with an unknown gene mutation.[13]

   a. Genetic testing should be recommended to individuals and families with a three-generation family history, a first-degree relative with known HNPCC, and/or those meeting the Amsterdam or Bethesda Criteria.

b. Genetic testing could provide a person with individualized risk avoidance, surveillance, and therapeutic options.

3. Penetrance, the likelihood that a disease will develop when a given mutation is present, is estimated in HNPCC.[12,13]

a. Risk of developing CRC before the age of 70 is 70–80%; general population risk is 2%.[12]

b. Risk of endometrial cancer in women before the age of 70 is 42–60%; general population risk is 1.5%.[12]

c. The risk of CRC or endometrial cancer developing before the age of 50 is 20–25%; general population risk is 0.2%.[12]

d. The risk of developing a second cancer within 15 years of the initial cancer diagnosis is 50%.[12]

❖ The Amsterdam Criteria-II, also known as the 1, 2, 3 Rule, helps identify families at risk of CRC.[12]

1 or more family members with CRC diagnosed before age 50 AND
2 or more generations affected by CRC AND
3 or more relatives with verified HNPCC-associated cancer (CRC, endometrial, small bowel, ureter, or renal cancers), one of which

must be a first-degree relative of the other two members

❖ The Bethesda Criteria are clinicopathologic criteria that may identify individuals at highest risk of HNPCC (only one criteria is needed).[12]

1. Individuals whose families meet Amsterdam Criteria
2. Individuals with two HNPCC-related cancers—colonic or associated extracolonic
3. Individuals with CRC plus a first-degree relative with CRC and/or HNPCC-related associated extracolonic cancer, and/or colorectal adenoma (diagnosed before age 40); one of the cancers must have been diagnosed before age 45.
4. Individuals with CRC or endometrial cancer diagnosed before the age of 45
5. Individuals with a right-sided CRC (undifferentiated or poorly differentiated pattern [solid/cribiform characteristics]) diagnosed before the age of 45
6. Individuals with a signet-ring cell CRC diagnosed before the age of 45
7. Individuals diagnosed before the age of 40 with colorectal adenomas

❖ Screening recommendations for these high-risk families are outlined in Chapter 3, Table 3–3.[12]

❖ Recommended management involves a segmental colectomy with continued close monitoring for second cancers—colon or extracolonic.

Intestinal Conditions

❖ Comorbid conditions of the bowel put individuals at an increased risk of CRC.

  ❖ Inflammatory bowel disease, e.g., ulcerative colitis, and Crohn's disease are associated with a 30-fold increased risk of CRC.
  ❖ With colitis, the duration of active disease and the extent of dysplasia are factors.[1]

    1. The risk is cumulative and the percentage increases exponentially with each decade; 3% at 10 years after diagnosis to greater than 30% after 30 years with the disease.[1]
    2. The risk of CRC associated with Crohn's disease is higher than the general population, but less than with colitis. The risk is increased about 1.5 to 2 times.[1,9]

Environmental and Lifestyle Factors

❖ Environmental and lifestyle factors such as nutrition, alcohol intake, sedentary lifestyle, and cigarette smoking are implicated in the development of CRC.

❖ People cannot change their genes, but they can influence their environment and lifestyle to decrease their risk of developing cancer in general, and CRC in particular.

❖ Environmental factors

* Socioeconomic status does not directly play a role in CRC risk predisposition.
* Geography—The increased number of CRC cases in specific areas implicates geography, i.e., living in industrialized areas.
* The current geographic location is more reflective of increased risk than country of origin. That is, people relocating from an area of low risk to one of high risk increase their risk of CRC.[9] Key facets include embracing the lifestyle and diet of the new area.[7]
* With the exception of exposure to asbestos (increased risk of 1.5 to 2 times), there is no link to occupational exposures.[9]

❖ Lifestyle factors

* The association between lifestyle factors and the risk of CRC is often controversial and confusing to the public; research is ongoing.
* Diet
    1. Diets rich in animal fats and red meat have been linked in most studies to the development of CRC.[9]
    2. The risk to people who consume diets high in animal fat or red meat is 2 to 2.5 times higher than those who consume diets low in animal sources of meat.[15]
    3. Though animal fat has been implicated, the risk may be associated with total fat intake

rather than with the specific type of fat consumed.[15]

4. Fats in whole milk, margarines, salad oils, mayonnaise products, and fried foods are also major sources of fat.[15]

5. Though controversial, current research has not specifically supported the protective effect of fiber, yellow and green vegetables, or fruits.[1]

6. Research has supported the protective effect of calcium salts, calcium-rich foods, and folic acid.[1]

❖ Alcohol consumption

1. With the exception of a link between beer consumption and the development of rectal cancer, the relationship between alcohol consumption and colon cancer is inconsistent.[9]

❖ Cigarette smoking

1. Though the mechanism is not clear, there is a strong association between cigarette smoking and the development of gastrointestinal cancers, including CRC.[16]

2. Individuals who smoked for ≤ 20 years are 3 times more likely to have small adenomas, while those who've smoked for more than 20 years are 2.5 times more likely to have large adenomas.[9]

3. Though further research is needed, a recent report has suggested cigarette smoking may

cause microsatellite insufficiency (MSI), which plays a role in carcinogenesis.[17]

❖ Obesity and physical activity

1. Though the direct effect is unclear, obesity is associated with an increased risk of CRC.[18,19]

2. Regular activity/exercise reportedly decreases the risk of CRC.[18,19]

❖ Aspirin, nonsteriodal anti-inflammatory agents, cyclooxygenase-2 (COX-2) inhibitors, and hormone-replacement therapy

1. Observational studies have supported the use of aspirin and nonsteriodal agents to reduce the risk of polyp development, cancer incidence, and cancer mortality even though the exact dose and duration are unclear.[1]

2. COX-2 inhibitors may have a role in chemoprevention.

   a. The COX-2 inhibitor, celecoxib, is approved by the Food and Drug Administration (FDA) as part of the standard therapy to prevent polyp formation in patients with FAP

   b. The role of COX-2 inhibitors in preventing sporadic adenomas and CRC is under investigation

3. Hormone-replacement therapy is associated with a reduced risk of CRC in women, though the exact mechanism is not understood[9]

Recommendations

❖ The key is to "take action" (see Figure 2-1) and to be consistent and persistent with lifestyle changes

❖ With CRC evolving over the course of decades, there is time to incorporate lifestyle changes and reduce the risk of CRC

❖ Many of the recommended actions confer other health benefits, such as a decreased risk of heart disease, further justifying the changes

The Role of the Nurse

❖ Stay abreast of the data on risk predisposition and prevention

❖ Identify patients and families at high risk of developing CRC through careful family and medical history

❖ Refer individuals and families with an apparent genetic predisposition to a high-risk specialty clinic and/or a genetic counselor for further risk evaluation.

 ❖ Genetic counselors and nurses in genetic risk clinics should:

  1. Carefully evaluate a family history with several generations of CRC or extracolonic cancers
  2. Provide risk counseling and education so the individual and/or family can make an informed decision

FIGURE 2-1
Fast facts that could save your life

Second most common cancer

- Colorectal cancer is cancer of the colon or rectum.
- 148,300 people will be stricken this year[2]
- 56,600 people will die this year because of it[2]
- 90% of people with colorectal cancer are more than 50 years old
- Increased incidence above age 40
- Highest incidence is between the ages of 65 and 74

Colorectal cancer affects us all.

- Young people believe that it is a disease of the elderly
- Women believe that only men get it
- African Americans believe only whites get it
- Everyone believes that there is nothing you can do about it

Risk factors include:

- Age
- Diet high in animal fats and processed meat, low in fruits and vegetables
- Personal history of colorectal cancer, polyps, ulcerative colitis, or Crohn's disease
- Family history of colorectal cancer, polyps, or other cancers, e.g., breast, ovarian, or uterine
- Sedentary lifestyle

Take action!

- Exercise regularly
- Keep weight at recommended levels
- Eat less red meat
- Eat more fruits and vegetables (5–6 servings each day)
- Take a multivitamin with folic acid and calcium
- Don't smoke
- Limit alcohol
- Consider daily dose of aspirin, NSAIDs, or COX2 inhibitor, if approved by your doctor.

FIGURE 2–1
(continued)

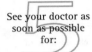

See your doctor as soon as possible for:

- Rectal bleeding
- Blood in your stool
- Abdominal cramping or pain
- Change in bowel habits lasting more than a few days
- Narrowing of the stool (ribbon-like)
- Weakness or fatigue
- Urge to have a bowel movement, even after just having one

Get checked!

- All men and women aged 50 or older should be screened.
- Don't wait for your doctor to recommend screening; tell him/her *you* want it!
- Starting at age 50, stool blood test every year
- Starting at age 50, flexible sigmoidoscopy every 5 years,

  or

- Starting at age 50, colonoscopy every 10 years
- Earlier and more frequent screening tests if family history of cancer at a young age

---

    3. Ensure patient confidentiality

    4. Assist in the decision-making process after positive genetic testing

❖ Educate patients and their families about recommended dietary modification to reduce their risk of CRC.

❖ Utilize risk assessment tools such as the risk assessment pathway noted in Figure 2-2 and the Harvard Center for Cancer Prevention, "Your

FIGURE 2-2
Risk assessment pathway

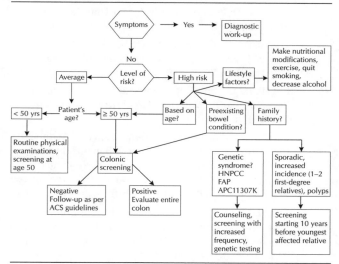

Source: Data from Saddler DA, Ellis C. "Colorectal Cancer." *Semin Oncol Nurs.* 1999; 15(1): 58–69.

Cancer Risk,™" available at
www.yourcancerrisk.harvard.edu.

❖ Because we all have some risk of developing CRC,
we should pay attention to the recommendations
and make changes to decrease that risk (Figure 2-1).

References

1. Ellenhorn JDI, Coia LR, Alberts SR, and Hoff PM.
"Colorectal and Anal Cancers." In Pazdur R, Coia LR,
Hoskins HJ, and Wagman LD, eds. *Cancer*

Management: A Multidisciplinary Approach, 6th edition. Melville, NY: PRR, Inc, 2002: 295–318.

2. Jemal A, Thomas A, Murray T, and Thun M. "Cancer Statistics, 2002." *CA Cancer J Clin.* 2002; 52(1): 23–47.

3. Jessup JM, McGinnis LS, Steele GD, *et al.* "The National Cancer Data Base Report on Colon Cancer." *Cancer.* 1996; 78: 918–926.

4. Engelking C. "Profiling Colorectal Cancer: Nature and Scope of the Disease." *Dev Supportive Cancer Care.* 1997; 1(2): 1–40.

5. Sargent D, Goldberg R, MacDonald J, *et al.* "Adjuvant Chemotherapy for Colon Cancer Is Beneficial without Significantly Increased Toxicity in Elderly Patients: Results from 3351 Patient Meta-analysis." *Proc Am Soc Clin Oncol.* 2000; 19:933 (abstr).

6. Saltz LB, Cox JV, Blanke C, *et al.*, for the Irinotecan Study Group. "Irinotecan Plus Fluorouracil and Leucovorin for Metastatic Colorectal Cancer." *N Engl J Med.* 2000; 343(13): 905–914.

7. Grobovsky L, Kaplon M, Krozer-Hamati A, *et al.* "Features of Cancer in Frail Elderly Patients (≥ 85 years of age)." *Proc Am Soc Clin Oncol.* 2000; 19:2469 (abstr).

8. Dadoly AM. "Moving into the Spotlight." *Harvard Pilgrim Health Care* Your Health. 2000; (Fall): 8–12.

9. Goldberg RM. "Gastrointestinal Tract Cancers." In Casciato DA, and Lowitz BB, eds. *Manual of Clinical Oncology,*.4th ed. Philadelphia, PA: Lippincott Williams & Wilkins, 2000: 182–194.

10. Greenlee RT, Murray T, Bolden S, *et al.* "Cancer Statistics, 2000." *CA Cancer J Clin.* 2000; 50(1): 7–33.

11. Houlston RS, Murday V, Harocopos C, *et al.* "Screening and Genetic Counseling for Relatives of

Patients with Colorectal Cancer in a Family Cancer Clinic. *BMJ*. 1990; 301(6748): 366–368.

12. American Medical Association (AMA) and the American Gastroenterological Association AGA). *Identifying and Managing Risks for Hereditary Nonpolyposis Colorectal Cancer and Endometrial Cancer (HNPCC)*. Chicago, IL: AMA, 2001.

13. Read TE. "Colorectal Cancer: Risk Factors and Recommendations for Early Detection." *Am Fam Physician*. June 1999. Available at http://www.findarticles.com/cf-0/m3225/11-59/55391765/print.jhtml. Accessed January 7, 2001.

14. Molecular Genetics Laboratory of John Hopkins Oncology Center. "APCI1307K." Available at http://www.coloncancer.org/HCCR-files/i1307k.htm. Accessed June 26, 2002.

15. Clifford C, Ballard-Barbash R, Lanza E, *et al.* "Diet and Cancer Risk." In Harras A, Edwards BK, Blot WJ, *et al.*, eds. *Cancer Rates and Risks*, 4th ed. NIH Pub. No. 96–691. Bethesda, MD: National Cancer Institute, 1996: 73–76.

16. Shopland DR. "Cigarette Smoking as a Cause of Cancer." In Harras A, Edwards BK, Blot WJ, *et al.*, eds. *Cancer Rates and Risks*, 4th ed. NIH Pub. No. 96–691. Bethesda, MD: National Cancer Institute, 1996: 67–72.

17. Neugut AI, Terry MB. "Cigarette Smoking and Microsatellite Instability: Causal Pathway or Marker-Defined Subset of Colon Tumors?" *J Natl Cancer Inst.* 2000; 92: 1791–1793.

18. Giovannucci E, Ascherio A, Rimm EB, *et al.* "Physical Activity, Obesity, and Risk for Colon Cancer and Adenoma in Men." *Ann Intern Med.* 1995; 122: 327–334.

19. Giovannucci E, Colditz GA, Stampfer MJ, *et al.* "Physical Activity, Obesity, and Risk for Colorectal Adenoma in Women." *Cancer Causes Control,* 1996; 7: 253–263.

20. Saddler DA, Ellis C. "Colorectal Cancer." *Semin Oncol Nurs.* 1999; 15 (1): 58–69.

3

Screening and Early Detection Guidelines

Introduction

Screening is justified when a disease is common, associated with significant morbidity or mortality, and there are affordable, accurate tests to detect the disease at an early stage.[1] In addition, the benefits of screening must outweigh the potential risks and/or costs. CRC affects over 130,000 people each year and more than half of them will die. It is estimated that approximately 20,000 to 30,000 lives could be saved if widespread screening and early detection methods were instituted.[2] The principles of CRC screening are to distinguish those likely to get cancer from those who will not. The goal of early detection is to diagnosis CRC while the tumor is small and potentially curable. The currently available screening tests differ in technical ability, sensitivity, cost, and risk, but all have compelling data that support their effectiveness while being cost effective.

Six Key Messages[3]

❖ CRC is preventable.

❖ Screening reduces CRC incidence and mortality.

❖ At age 50 all men and women should begin regular screening.

❖ High-risk individuals should begin screening earlier.

❖ Screening options are available; NOT screening is an unhealthy option.

❖ Screening is not a one time procedure, but rather an ongoing commitment to health.

Common Screening Methods

❖ Digital rectal examination (DRE)

❖ Fecal occult blood test (FOBT)

❖ Endoscopic visualization methods
  • Flexible sigmoidoscopy
  • Colonoscopy

❖ Double contrast barium enema (DCBE)

❖ Figure 3-1 illustrates the limitations of screening evaluations for colorectal cancer.[4]

Digital Rectal Examinations

❖ Benefits
  • DRE is a relatively painless, simple examination that can be done in the doctor's office without prior preparation.

FIGURE 3-1
Limitations of screening evaluations for colorectal cancer

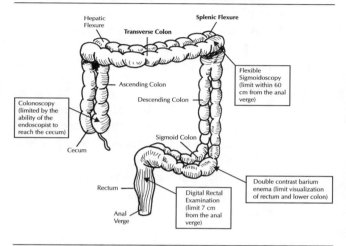

Source: Data from Ellis C, Saddler D. "Colorectal Cancer." In Yarbro CH, Frogge MH, Goodman M, *et al.*, eds. *Cancer Nursing: Principles and Practice,* 5th ed. Boston, MA: Jones and Bartlett Publishers, 2000: 1117–1137.

- ❖ Is useful to find masses in the anorectum (within reach of the examiner's digit)
- ❖ DRE should be performed in conjunction with other tests; i.e., sigmoidoscopy, colonoscopy, and DCBE.

❖ Limitations
- ❖ Fewer than 10% of rectal cancers and no colon cancers are within its limited reach, therefore, poor sensitivity for CRC.[1]

* Not recommended as the only screening method
* No data suggesting that DRE decreases the mortality rate of colon or rectal cancer
* Is less sensitive and specific than home FOBT[3]

Fecal Occult Blood Testing

❖ Benefits

* An effective screening method that reduces incidence by 20% and mortality by one third when repeated yearly;[5] annual screening is better than biennial screening.[3]
* A noninvasive test that detects blood in a sample of stool; it is recommended that the testing be done on stool from multiple bowel movements.
* The test is inexpensive–$10 to $25.[3]
* The compliance rate is better than with other more invasive tests though compliance is still an issue.
* No special training is required and most samples are processed in the physician's office.

❖ Limitations

* It does not detect tumors in the rectosigmoid colon.
* Patients need clear instructions–sample collection and dietary and medication restrictions. When patients receive good instructions, they are more likely to follow through.[3]
* Some CRC tumors do not bleed at all; many do not bleed until the later stages, or bleeding may

only be intermittent, therefore the lesions may not be detected.

❖ If the specimen card is not brought in quickly for testing (<7 days), it can affect the outcome.

❖ Procedure: Two samples are taken from three consecutive stools. Each sample is placed on the testing card. Patients should not ingest anti-inflammatory drugs or aspirin (> than one adult aspirin/day) for 7 days prior to testing; vitamin C at doses >250mg from supplements or citrus fruits and juices for 3 days prior to testing; or red meat, turnips, and horseradish for 2 days prior to testing.[3]

❖ Available guiac-based tests[3]

❖ The Hemoccult/Hemoccult II Test

1. Only test shown effective in clinical trials[3]
2. Test is performed in the physician's office.

❖ Hemoccult Sensa

1. Sensitivity and specificity are similar to the rehydrated methods.
2. Test is performed in the physician's office.

❖ HemeSelect

1. New immunochemical test specific for hemoglobin may decrease the rate of false positives.
2. Currently testing is done in a laboratory.

Sigmoidoscopy

❖ Benefits

   ❖ Allows direct visualization of the rectum, the sigmoid, and the descending colon

      1. The rigid sigmoidoscope reaches to about 30 cm in length.
      2. The flexible sigmoidoscope reaches to about 60 cm in length and offers a better view of the lower bowel.

   ❖ When it reaches the splenic flexure, sigmoidoscopy is 80% accurate in diagnosing significant tumors throughout the colon, primarily because 50% of lesions are located in the distal colon. A positive sigmoidoscopy then leads to a colonoscopy and thus an examination of the whole colon.[6]

   ❖ Cost is approximately $150 to $300.[3]

❖ Limitations

   ❖ Must be performed by a trained examiner, though this can include trained primary care providers and nurses

   ❖ Bowel preparation is required: two or more cleansing enemas the morning of the test.

   ❖ Complications include bowel perforation.

   ❖ Case control studies have shown a benefit in lowering incidence and mortality of CRC.[7]

1. Two clinical trials are underway to evaluate the effectiveness of flexible sigmoidoscopy, but the data are not expected until 2008.[7]

❖ Procedure

  ❖ The test is usually done in a doctor's office without sedation and takes 10 to 20 minutes.[3]
  ❖ Patients are positioned on their left side with knees bent to their chest. After being lubricated, the sigmoidoscope is inserted into the anus and passed up toward the splenic flexure. Patients may notice some discomfort, e.g., spasms or transient need to move their bowels as the tube is inserted and advanced or cramping as air is inserted into the bowel to allow the physician a better view of the colon. Suction is used to remove stool or secretions in the bowel to improve visualization.
  ❖ Polyps are usually biopsied and excised. Individuals with large or multiple polyps are referred for a colonoscopy, because there is an increased risk of more polyps beyond the reach of the sigmoidoscope and larger polyps are more likely to be malignant.
  ❖ Postprocedure considerations
    1. There may be some flatus, and if a biopsy was taken, some blood may be noted in the stool.
    2. Patients do not need transportation assistance and can resume regular activities immediately.

Colonoscopy

❖ Benefits

- ❖ Offers complete direct visualization of the entire colon in addition to therapeutic abilities.
- ❖ Reduction in incidence and mortality of CRC established indirectly; observational studies demonstrate a 75% to 90% reduction in new CRC by colonoscopic exam and the removal of polyps.[8] In addition, the detection and removal of early cancers lowers the mortality rate.[2]
- ❖ Considered to be the most accurate screening measure and is considered the standard method.[7]

❖ Limitations

- ❖ A full-bowel preparation with an oral cathartic solution, laxatives, and/or enemas are required as a clean colon is absolutely necessary.
- ❖ Patients at risk for endocarditis should receive prophylactic antibiotics.
- ❖ Complications during the procedure: side effects from sedation and bowel perforation (e.g., malaise, bleeding, abdominal pain and distention, fever, and mucopurulent drainage)
- ❖ Cost ($800 to $1600) is considered high and is not reimbursed by all health insurance providers.[3]
- ❖ Requires trained endoscopists and endoscopy suites and equipment, which at this time are limited in availability in many areas.
- ❖ May miss lesions in blind corners, mucosal folds, and in the cecum if it is not reached.[6]

❖ Procedure

  ❖ Bowel preparation: clear liquid diet for 48 hours prior to the exam; drink either 10 oz. of magnesium citrate or 1 gallon of Go-Lytely as prescribed.

  ❖ Procedure usually takes 30–45 minutes.[3]

  ❖ Upon arriving at the hospital, patients are medicated with either an intramuscular or intravenous injection of a sedative of the doctors' choosing. The sedative decreases the discomfort caused by the length of the colonoscope, the distension of the colon with air, and the duration of the procedure.

  ❖ Patients are positioned on their left side with knees bent to their chest. After being lubricated, the colonoscope is inserted into the anus, advanced into the sigmoid colon, through the splenic flexure, along the transverse colon, through the hepatic flexure, and into the ascending colon and cecum. The insertion of the tube may be uncomfortable, e.g., patients may experience a transient need to move their bowels as the tube is manipulated or cramping as air is inserted into the bowel to allow better view of the colon. During the exam, suction is used to remove blood or secretions that can obscure visualization of the colonic lining.

  ❖ Forceps and/or a cytology brush are passed through the core of the colonoscope to biopsy and excise polyps and/or lesions.

* When patients are alert, vital signs are stable, and there are no postprocedure complications, they can be discharged home.
* Postprocedure considerations—patients usually:[3]
  1. Miss work for 1 day
  2. Require a ride home afterwards
  3. Pass large amounts of flatus
  4. Note blood in their stool if a polyp was removed
  5. Resume their usual diet

Barium Enema

* Radiologic examination of the entire colon defining contours in colonic lining

* Two methods to perform a barium enema
  * Single contrast study with barium alone
  * Double contrast study with air instilled into the colon after the barium has been instilled; the double contrast method is preferred for screening as it provides better delineation of polyps.

* Benefits
  * Procedure takes 20–30 minutes and is performed without sedation.[3]
  * Is less expensive than colonoscopy and is considered a cost-effective method to find larger lesions
  * Cost is approximately $250 to $500.[3]

❖ Limitations

❖ An experienced radiologist is required to perform and interpret the test.

❖ Bowel preparation is required; clear liquid diet, laxatives, and enemas during the 24 hours prior to the examination.

❖ Inadequate bowel preparation will impair the quality of the radiographic pictures.[9]

❖ Barium swallow within several days before a barium enema is contraindicated, as it will impair the quality of the subsequent films.[9]

❖ If the patient is unable to retain the barium, the test will be incomplete.[9]

❖ DCBE offers only evaluation; it does not offer therapeutic capabilities. Therefore, if a lesion or adenoma is seen, a colonoscopy will be needed, putting the patient through a second procedure.

❖ There is no data confirming that DCBE decreases the mortality rate of CRC cancer.

1. The sensitivity of DCBE varies by the size of the polyp, i.e., it is more sensitive at detecting polyps larger than 1 cm.[1] It is less sensitive at detecting smaller than 1 cm lesions than colonoscopy.[7]

2. The false-negative rate ranges from 2% to 61% due to poor bowel preparation, misinterpretation of results, and difficulties identifying small lesions.[6]

❖ Procedure

   ❖ An antispasmodic may be given prior to the procedure. Patients lie prone with a flexible 2 cm tube inserted into the rectum as the liquid barium is instilled. The patient must change position to advance the barium, turning first to the left side, and then right side, then the table is tilted to a standing position to fill the bowel as far as the cecum. The progression of the barium is monitored by fluoroscopy. Air is instilled into the colon to assist with the progression of the barium and to "press" the barium towards the colon wall to improve definition of the mucosa. There may be some discomfort as the patient changes position with the barium tube in place and if air is instilled too quickly.

   ❖ Radiographs outlining the bowel are taken once the barium has advanced to the desired location, ideally to the cecum. Patients can leave the hospital immediately after the examination.

   ❖ Postprocedure considerations

     1. Patients can return to work after the procedure, but they will pass barium frequently for a few days after the examination.

     2. Constipation is common; therefore, patients should drink a lot of fluids and may need a prescription for a stool softener or laxative.

Controversies

❖ There are many controversies over which screening methods to use for CRC.

❖ FOBT controversies

  ❖ False-negative and false-positive results are reported.

  ❖ FOBT significantly reduces the mortality rate but does not improve overall survival possibly due to comorbid conditions in those screened.

  ❖ It is controversial as to which FOBT kit to use— a rehydrated one, nonhydrated kit, or the newer hemoglobin immunoassay kit that reportedly decreases the rate of false positives.

❖ DCBE controversies

  ❖ 5–15% will have a positive test and require a follow-up colonoscopy.[3]

  ❖ Variable quality of the test across the country[3]

  ❖ Small adenomas have a low risk of malignant transformation before the next examination and could therefore be left in place. Dilemma: Adenomas smaller than 1 cm carry less than a 1% risk of becoming cancerous, but small adenomas with villous elements have a 10% increase risk and should be removed.[10]

❖ Sigmoidoscopy controversies

  ❖ It is better than the FOBT at detecting small polyps and gives fewer false positives, but overall has low sensitivity for detecting adenomas less than 1 cm.

- ❖ Controversy about who should biopsy polyps—primary care provider or a specialist
- ❖ Sigmoidoscopy detects cancers and polyps in the left colon, but it does not visualize the entire colon.
- ❖ With a reported increase in adenomas proximal to the splenic flexure, it is important to examine this area, but such lesions would be out of reach of the sigmoidoscope. Therefore, screening sigmoidoscopy for CRC has been compared to doing a screening mammogram on only one breast. Hence, the argument is made in favor of colonoscopy that examines the whole colon.
- ❖ About 5% to 15% of examinations require follow up with a colonoscopy.[3]

- ❖ Colonoscopy controversies
  - ❖ Colonoscopies are expensive, ranging from $800 to $1600 and many insurance carriers do not cover the cost. The cost may decrease with increased availability and lower procedure costs.[3]
  - ❖ It views the entire colon and has therapeutic capabilities, but has higher complication rates and the patient needs to be sedated.
  - ❖ There are a limited number of endoscopists.
  - ❖ Role and competition issues are obstacles for training other healthcare providers.
  - ❖ There can be a long wait for a screening colonoscopy, but if this method becomes the national screening standard, there could be a significant shortage.

- Hence, the controversy surrounds using this examination for the average-risk individual without symptoms, though there is consensus in using it for moderate to high-risk individuals.
- Cost effectiveness of screening modalities is often debated due to cost constraints on health-care dollars.
  - Issues include the appropriate age to initiate screening, the method used, and cost-benefit analyses.[11-13]
  - Colorectal screening for the average-risk person would cost $15,000 to $20,000 per year of life saved. *Note:* none of the individual methodologies cost more than that.
  - This is considered very cost effective based on the federal government's benchmark of $40,000 per year of life saved (*Note:* mammography costs $37,000 per year of life saved).[12,13]
- Possible solutions to the controversy
  - Risk and/or targeted age algorithms could help guide only those individuals in most need of a colonoscopy towards that procedure.
  - If there was a positive FOBT in an average-risk individual, the primary provider could order either a colonsocopy or a DCBE with a flexible sigmoidoscopy as a low-cost alternative to the patient.[7]
  - No single test is without controversy for CRC screening; therefore, an informed shared decision between the physician and individual should be made based on risk factors.

❖ The only unacceptable answer is no screening.

Who Should Be Screened for CRC?

Individuals must share their family history and
known risk factors with their primary care provider
to accurately assess their level of risk[14]

❖ Average risk individuals[7]
  ❖ All men and women over the age of 50,
    regardless of race or ethnic background—Note
    Table 3-1 for screening recommendations.

❖ Moderate risk individuals[7]
  ❖ Those with a personal or family history of
    adenomatous polyps or CRC—Women with a
    family history of breast, ovarian, or
    endometrial cancer, but without a specific
    genetic syndrome are also at increased risk.
    Note Table 3-2 for screening recommendations.

❖ High risk individuals[7]
  ❖ Those with current or preexisting bowel
    conditions (inflammatory bowel disease,
    ulcerative colitis, and Crohn's disease) are
    considered at high risk while those with
    hereditary syndromes such as FAP or HNPCC
    are considered at very high risk.[7] Note Table 3-3
    for screening recommendations.

❖ Estimates are that average-risk individuals
  account for approximately 70% to 80% of new
  CRC cases, moderate-risk individuals account for
  approximately 15% to 20% of the cases, and only
  5% to 10% are from high-risk individuals.[1]

TABLE 3-1
Screening Recommendations Men and Women Age 50 and Older at Average Risk for Colorectal Cancer

Procedure: Choice of One of the Following	Interval After Initiated at Age 50	Comments
Fecal Occult Blood Test (FOBT) OR	Every year	Procedure: 2 samples from 3 consecutive bowel movements obtained at home; tested by physician
Flexible Sigmoidoscopy OR	Every 5 years	
FOBT plus Flexible Sigmoidoscopy OR	FOBT every year; Flexible Sigmoidoscopy every 5 years	Procedure for FOBT as above. This combination is preferred over either test alone.[7]
Double Contrast Barium Enema OR	Every 5 years	
Colonoscopy	Every 10 years	

Note: For any positive result from FOBT, flexible sigmoidoscopy, or DCBE, a colonoscopy is recommended. Continued surveillance is then determined based on those results.

Note: An alternative to colonoscopy is the combination of DCBE and flexible sigmoidoscopy, but if those are positive, a colonoscopy is recommended.

Sources: American Cancer Society (2001) and the U.S. Preventive Services Task Force (1996).[7,16]

TABLE 3-2
Screening Recommendations Men and Women at Increased Risk for Colorectal Cancer

Population	Age to Start Screening	Recommended Procedure	Comments
Individuals with single, <1 cm polyp	3 to 6 years after removal of polyp	Colonoscopy	If test is negative, can then be screened per average risk. Alternative strategy: double contrast barium enema alone or with flexible sigmoidoscopy.
Individuals with >1 cm polyp, multiple polyps, or polyps with dysplasia or villous changes	Within 3 years after removal of polyp	Colonoscopy	If first test is negative, repeat in 3 years. If second test is negative, then screen as average risk. Alternate strategy as above.
Individuals with a personal history of resected colorectal cancer (CRC)	Within 1 year after surgery	Colonoscopy	If first test is negative, repeat in 3 years. If second test is negative repeat every 5 years. Alternate strategy as above.

(continued)

TABLE 3-2
Screening Recommendations Men and Women at Increased Risk for Colorectal Cancer (continued)

Population	Age to Start Screening	Recommended Procedure	Comments
Individual with first-degree relative diagnosed with polyps or CRC before the age of 60, or multiple first-degree relatives diagnosed at any age with polyps or CRC (no hereditary syndromes)	Age 40, or 10 years less than the youngest affected relative, whichever is earlier	Colonoscopy	Every 5–10 years. Alternate strategy as above.

Sources: American Cancer Society (2001) and the U.S. Preventive Services Task Force (1996).[7,16]

TABLE 3-3
Screening Recommendations Men and Women at High Risk for Colorectal Cancer

Population	Age to Start Screening	Recommended Procedure and Frequency	Comments
Familial Adenomatous Polyposis (FAP)	Puberty	Endoscopy every 1–2 years and genetic counseling	Consider genetic testing. If positive, recommended management is colectomy. Consider referral to experienced FAP clinic.
Hereditary Nonpolyposis Colon Cancer	Age 20–25	Colonoscopy every 1–2 years.	Consider genetic testing. If not tested or if positive, repeat colonoscopy every 1–2 years until age 40, then repeat yearly.
	Age 30–35	Gastroscopy, ultrasound, and urine cytology every 1–2 years.	Consider referral to experienced HNPCC clinic.
	Age 20–25	For women, gynecologic exam, transvaginal ultrasound, CA-125 every 1–2 years	
		Genetic counseling	

(continued)

TABLE 3-3
Screening Recommendations Men and Women at High Risk for Colorectal Cancer (continued)

Population	Age to Start Screening	Recommended Procedure and Frequency	Comments
Inflammatory bowel disease, Chronic ulcerative colitis, Crohn's disease	Within 8 years after onset of pancolitis or within 12–15 years after start of left-sided colitis	Colonoscopy every 1–2 years	Recommend biopsy of dysplastic areas. The extent and duration of the disease are factors used to determine need for a colectomy.

Consider referral to experience high-risk clinic. |

Sources: American Cancer Society (2001), the U.S. Preventive Services Task Force (1996), and the American Medical Association/American Gastroenterological Association (2001).[7,16,17]

Screening Recommendations

❖ Several organizations have established screening guidelines for CRC. Though they are somewhat different in terms of specific details, there are several important common details.[7]

  ❖ All are evidence-based.
  ❖ All offer a selection of options.
  ❖ All encourage shared decision making between physician and patient.
  ❖ All recommend screening for average-risk individuals starting at the age of 50.
  ❖ All acknowledge that any of the screening options are better than no screening at all.

❖ Despite the current body of knowledge supporting the benefits of CRC screening (decrease in both incidence and mortality), the majority of Americans are **not** being screened.

  ❖ Of those 50 years of age or older, 19% had had an FOBT within the last year and 32.3% had undergone either a sigmoidoscopy or colonoscopy within the last 5 years.[15] Men are more likely to have an endoscopic exam (34.2% men versus 17.1% women), while women are more likely to have had an FOBT (21.3% men versus 30.3% women). (*Note:* This compares to 63% of women having mammograms and 89% having pap tests.) White Americans are most likely to be screened, followed in descending order by Asian/Pacific Islanders, African

Americans, American Indian/Alaska Native, and Hispanics.[15]

❖ Shared decision making, where the individual is told about each screening option in detail—the accuracy, cost, potential for prevention, discomforts, and complications—is highly recommended. Individuals can then select a screening method based on personal risks, preferences, cost, feasibility, capacity to endure any of the discomforts or complications, and local availability of trained examiners.

❖ Tables 3-1, 3-2, and 3-3 outline the current screening recommendations.[7,16,17]

When to Stop Screening[16]

❖ There is little evidence of a specific age at which screening should be stopped.

❖ Inference could be made that with a decrease in CRC incidence after the 8th decade of life that screening could be stopped once the individuals are in their 80s.

❖ Unless there are significant comorbid conditions that would prohibit treatment, screening would likely be a benefit and should be continued.

Barriers to Screening[3]

If screening works, why aren't more people doing it?

❖ Screening compliance rates are influenced by many factors.

* Lack of public awareness about CRC and about the benefits of regular screening
* Lack of professional awareness about CRC screening guidelines, leading to no or inconsistent recommendation for screening
* Assumption by healthcare providers that a DRE in the office is sufficient to screen for CRC
* Limited time and staff to explain CRC screening tests, among all the other preventative care recommendations, to patients during routine clinic visits
* Patients' unclear understanding about the tests, the meaning of a positive test, and what is required to investigate a positive result
* Inconsistent referral of positive results to a gastroenterologist
* No reminder system in the office to prompt the healthcare provider about prevention guidelines and CRC screening in particular[18]
* Lack of preparedness of primary healthcare providers to offer screening tests
* Limited availability of trained endoscopists, endoscopy suites, and equipment resulting in a long lag time for an appointment
* Uncertainty among consumers about insurance benefits
* Inability of consumers to pay for the cost of screening tests
* Lack of coverage for most screening methods by third-party payers and health maintenance. Medicare covers FOBT and helps pay for

flexible sigmoidoscopy, DCBE, and colonoscopy. *Note:* only physician providers are reimbursed for flexible sigmoidoscopy.
* Drawbacks of the screening options (e.g., false-positive and false-negative rates, negative perception of screening procedures (discomfort, embarrassment), fear of hearing the cancer diagnosis)
* Social stigma surrounding CRC
* Cultural barriers: fear of the medical community, disregard for the physicians' recommendations, and written material for screening tests in English only

What Can Be Done to Increase Screening?

* Develop educational programs and materials for patients, healthcare providers, managed care organizations, and government officials
    * Goal: increase awareness of the impact of CRC and of the value of screening and surveillance
    * Recommend multiple formats: videotapes, brochures, chart markers, symposia, print articles—public and professional articles—and media advertisements. Materials must be culturally and literacy sensitive.

* Change legislation to increase support for CRC screening

* Develop new screening tests that will be efficacious yet may be less offensive for the patient

Emerging Technologies

❖ Computed tomography colonography (also called CT colonography or virtual colonoscopy)[19]

  ❖ Uses magnetic resonance imaging (MRI) or computed tomography (CT) scan to make a computer-generated, three-dimensional image of the colon

  ❖ Because it is considered experimental, most insurance providers do not cover it.

  ❖ A complete colon preparation is still required; air is introduced into the colon so there is still some discomfort. Unlike traditional colonoscopy, it is not an invasive procedure and sedation is not needed. However, if a polyp is found, patients must undergo a traditional colonoscopy to biopsy and excise the polyp, thus requiring an additional bowel preparation and procedure.

❖ Molecular Screening of the Stool[20]

  ❖ These tests would assess for DNA, RNA, and/or protein marker abnormalities shed from precancerous polyps and cancerous tumors into the colon. These would be detected in the laboratory when the patient's stool was examined.

  ❖ No special diet, medication restrictions, or bowel preparations are required.

  ❖ These may improve compliance, though the patient still needs to handle their stool, which is often considered offensive. Another drawback is that even if these tests are positive, the cancer may be too small to be detected by current methods.

❖ The M2A Capsule Endoscope[21,22]

  ❖ The ingestible capsule holds a miniature video camera, light source, batteries, transmitter, and antenna—all disposable. It beams color pictures of the intestinal tract back to a receiver (an array of sensors) worn around the patient's waist. After fasting overnight, the patients swallow the grape-sized capsule and go about their daily activities. The system is noninvasive and painless. After a day or so, the physician downloads the pictures onto a portable data recorder and a computer workstation equipped with advanced image processing software. The patient excretes the capsule within 8 to 72 hours.[21,22]

  ❖ Efficacy is reported at 55% compared with 30% for traditional upper gastrointestinal enteroscopy.[21]

  ❖ Cost is $20,000 for the computer workstation and $450 per capsule.[21]

  ❖ At this time, the battery lasts 8 hours or less and therefore cannot be used to image the large bowel, though this may come in the future.

  ❖ The system is FDA approved for imaging of the UGI and small bowel.[21]

The Role of Nurses

❖ Conduct risk assessments on all patients, making sure all information is as complete and accurate as possible

❖ Educate patients about the epidemiology, risk factors, signs, and symptoms of CRC, and the importance of screening and early detection

❖ Recommend at least one screening option to all eligible patients

❖ Tutor individuals on ways to reduce their risk

❖ Develop screening programs

❖ Inform patients of screening clinics and the significance of detecting CRC early

❖ Refer appropriate individuals and families to genetic counselors for further assessment and/or genetic testing

❖ Refer appropriate and interested individuals to chemoprevention clinical trials

❖ Educate peers about CRC in general and screening and early detection methods in particular

❖ Participate in programs to impact government regulations supporting screening tests

❖ Advanced practice nurses may perform screening sigmoidoscopies, thereby taking an active role in primary and secondary prevention.

The Key Is Education

❖ Well-informed healthcare providers will recommend screening tests that will increase compliance by individuals.

❖ Well-informed patients are more likely to take responsibility for their well being and request screening tests if they are not offered.

❖ Well-informed government officials will influence change to the healthcare system in terms of screening and early detection.

References

1. Winawer S, Fletcher R, Miller L, *et al.* "Colorectal Screening: Clinical Guidelines and Rationale." *Gastroenterology.* 1997; 112: 594–641.

2. National Cancer Institute. *Conquering Colorectal Cancer: A Blueprint for the Future—The Report of the Colorectal Cancer Progress Review Group.* Bethesda, MD: National Cancer Institute, 2000.

3. Center for Disease Control. "A Call to Action: Prevention and Early Detection of Colorectal Cancer." November 5, 2001. Available at http://www.cdc.gov/cancer/colorctl/calltoaction/slide-index.htm. Accessed on July 12, 2002.

4. Ellis C, and Saddler D. "Colorectal Cancer." In Yarbro CH, Frogge MH, Goodman M, *et al. Cancer Nursing: Principles and Practice*, 5th ed. Boston, MA: Jones and Bartlett Publishers, 2000: 1117–1137.

5. Mandel JS, Bond JH, Church, *et al.* "Reducing Mortality from Colorectal Cancer Screening for Fecal Occult Blood. Minnesota Colon Cancer Control Study." [published erratum appears in *New England Journal of*

Medicine 1993 August 26; 329:672] *New England Journal of Medicine* 1993; 1365–1371.

6. Ellenhorn JDI, Coia LR, Alberts SR, and Hoff PM. "Colorectal and Anal Cancers." In Pazdur R, Coia LR, Hoskins HJ, and Wagman LD, eds. *Cancer Management: A Multidisciplinary Approach*, 6th ed. Melville, NY: PRR, Inc, 2002: 295–318.

7. American Cancer Society. "American Cancer Society Guidelines on Screening and Surveillance for the Early Detection of Adenomatous Polyps and Colorectal Cancer—Update 2001." *CA: A Cancer Journal for Clinicians*. January/February 2001. 51(1): 44–54.

8. Notice to Readers: National Colorectal Cancer Awareness Month—March 2000. Morbidity and Mortality Weekly Report; March 17, 2000. 49(10): 212.

9. *Contrast Radiography: Illustrated Guide to Diagnostic Testing*. Springhouse, PA, 1993: 841–843.

10. Bilhartz L, and Croft C. "Rational Approach to Colon Cancer Screening." In Bilhartz L, ed. *Gastrointestinal Disease in Primary Care*. New York: Lippincott Williams & Wilkins, 2000: 119–131.

11. Rosenblaum D, Shiff S. "Chemoprevention of Colorectal Cancer: A Practical Approach." *Prim Care Cancer*. 1999; 19(6), (suppl 3). Available at http://www.cancernetwork.com/home/frames.htm?http://www.cancernetwork.com/drugs/Maxipime.htm&3. Accessed July 12, 2002.

12. Costable J Jr, and Weissman G. "What the Primary-Care Physician Needs to Know About Sigmoidoscopy." *Prim Care Cancer*. 1999; 19(6). Available at http://www.cancernetwork.com/home/frames.htm?http://www.cancernetwork.com/drugs/Maxipime.htm&3. Accessed July 12, 2002.

13. "Colorectal Cancer Screening Is Cost-Effective OTA Study Shows." *Oncology*. 1996; 10(5). Available at

http://www.cancernetwork.com/home/frames.htm?http://www.cancernetwork.com/drugs/Maxipime.htm&3. Accessed July 12, 2002.

14. "New National Colorectal Cancer Practice Guidelines: Recommended Life Saving Tests." American Gastroenterology Association, 1997. Available at www.gastro.org/phys-sci/fact-sheets/newguidelines.html. Accessed November 16, 2000.

15. Smith RA, Cokkinides V, von Eschenback AC, Levin B, Cohen C, Runowicz C, Sener S Saslow D, and Eyre H. "American Cancer Society Guidelines for the Early Detection of Cancer." *CA: A Cancer Journal for Clinicians.* January/February 2002; 52 (1): 8–22.

16. United States Preventive Service Task Force. *Guide to Clinical Preventive Services,* 2nd ed. 1996. Available at www.ahrg.gov/clinic/cpsix.htm. Accessed July 12, 2002.

17. American Medical Association (AMA) and the American Gastroenterological Association (AGA). *Identifying and Managing Risks for Hereditary Nonpolyposis Colorectal Cancer and Endometrial Cancer (HNPCC).* Chicago, IL: AMA, 2001.

18. "Primary Care Physicians and Colon Cancer Screening: Not so Easy." *Prim Care Cancer.* 1999; 16(8). Available at http://intouch.cancernetwork.com/journals/primary/p9609d.htm. Accessed August 29, 2000.

19. Halligan S, and Fenlon HM. "Virtual Colonoscopy." *BMJ* 1999; 319: 1249–1252.

20. Taus M. "New Colon Cancer Test Developed." *Newsday.* 2000. Available at http://newsday.com/ap/health-science/ap545.htm. Accessed December 20, 2000.

21. WebMD. "FDA OKs Swallowed Camera-Pill That Looks for Bowel Problems." August 1, 2001. Available at http://content.health.msn.com/content/article/1728.85347. Accessed June 28, 2002.

22. Boone Hospital Center. "Expanding the Scope of GI." November 29, 2001. Available at www.boone.org/news/pillcam.html. Accessed June 28, 2002.

4

Emerging Prevention Strategies

Introduction

There is no one specific, proven method to prevent any cancer, let alone colorectal cancer (CRC). We can reduce our risk in a variety of ways. The majority of us can identify risk factors and control behaviors, especially lifestyle factors that contribute to the development of CRC. High-risk individuals may choose surgical options, chemoprevention agents, and/or increased surveillance. Chemoprevention agents are an important key for the future.

Definitions in Prevention

- ❖ Cancer prevention: all measures that limit the progression of cancer at any time during its course

- ❖ Primary cancer prevention: reducing the risk of cancer by avoiding known carcinogens to prevent the occurrence of cancer in healthy individuals[1]

- ❖ Secondary cancer prevention: define individuals and/or populations at increased risk for cancer and screen for precursor lesions in the absence of symptoms or detect cancers at early stages, when cure is more likely

❖ Tertiary cancer prevention: monitor for and prevent the recurrence of cancer to deter the progress of clinically overt cancer and to minimize morbidity by preventing complications from cancer[2]

Approaches to the Prevention of CRC

❖ Chemoprevention
  ❖ Vitamins, minerals, and antioxidants
  ❖ Aspirin, nonsteriodal anti-inflammatory agents, cyclooxygenese 2 inhibitors

❖ Prophylactic surgery

❖ Dietary modifications

❖ Lifestyle changes

Chemoprevention

❖ Definition: a pharmacologic intervention to reverse, suppress, or prevent the carcinogenic process from progressing to invasive cancer

❖ The multistep process of carcinogenesis supports the premise of chemoprevention.[2]

❖ Genetic mutations, accumulated over a period of 5- to 10+-years, cause normal mucosa to proceed from hyperplastic polyps to a dysplastic growth, to a cancerous tumor. This time frame means there are opportunities to intervene with chemopreventive agents and impact this natural process and prevent the malignant outcome.

❖ Probable mechanisms of action of chemopreventive agents

  ❖ Limit or prevent exposure of cells to tumor initiators or promoters
  ❖ Stimulate the inactivation and excretion of potential initiators or promoters
  ❖ Block the oncogene expression by inhibiting, modifying, or blocking the activation of proto-oncogenes[3]
  ❖ Regain control over cell replication and differentiation by inactivating tumor-suppressor genes

Vitamins, Minerals, and Antioxidants

❖ Vitamins and minerals exert their effect through a variety of means.

  ❖ Vitamins A, C, E, and beta-carotene have not shown a remarkable protective effect for CRC development.[4] Research on the benefit of selenium is inconsistent.[5] Therefore, there is no support at present for their use in CRC prevention.[4,6,7]
  ❖ Laboratory studies have suggested a preventative effect of calcium, observational studies have noted that persons with increased intake of vitamin D and calcium have a decreased risk of colon cancer, but human studies have shown little or no effect.[4]

1. More information is needed before calcium can be supported as a chemoprevention agent.[4]

❖ Epidemiology studies show an inverse relationship between folic acid and CRC though the mechanism for this association is debatable.[4]

1. Low folic acid levels are associated with higher frequency of CRC
2. High folic acid has been shown in some studies to substantially lower the risk of CRC, but more research is needed.[4]

❖ Aspirin, nonsteroidal anti-inflammatory drugs (NSAIDs), and cyclooxygenase 2 (COX2) inhibitors

❖ Aspirin and NSAIDs inhibit cylooxygenase (COX) and thereby affect prostaglandins, which modulate cell proliferation, tumor growth, and immune response. It is theorized that aspirin and NSAIDs inhibit both forms of cyclooxygenase: COX 1 and COX2. COX 1 produces prostaglandins that protect the GI tract, kidneys, and platelet aggregation. Side effects of aspirin and NSAIDs are felt to be due to the inhibition of COX1. COX2, which is primarily inducible, appears to play a role in mediating prostaglandins, which influence tumor promotion and inflammation. The anticarcinogenic effect of these agents is felt to be due to the inhibition of COX2.

❖ Observational studies have demonstrated that aspirin and NSAIDs can decrease the incidence of polyp formation, decrease the incidence of CRC, and reduce mortality.

❖ A recent randomized trial reported a 19% reduction in adenomas with low-dose aspirin (80 mg per day) though a higher dose of aspirin (325 mg per day) showed only a 4% reduction. Another study showed no aspirin effect compared with placebo.[4]

❖ In FAP, sulindac has demonstrated a 56% reduction in the number of polyps in one randomized, placebo-controlled study, but no effect in primary prevention of polyps in this population in another such study. The Food and Drug Administration (FDA) has not yet approved sulindac as a chemopreventive agent for FAP.[8]

❖ The National Cancer Institute (NCI) has an active chemoprevention program looking at aspirin and various NSAIDs, e.g., sulindac, piroxicam, ibuprofen, exisulind, and celecoxib. The endpoint is adenoma suppression, which the FDA has recommended as an endpoint for clinical trials.

1. Overall, research implies a potential role for aspirin and NSAIDs in the prevention of CRC incidence and mortality, but they are not yet recommended. More information is needed about the duration, dose, and side effects with long-term use.[4] In addition, it is not known if one NSAID is better than another one.

- ❖ Cyclooxygenase 2 (COX2) specific inhibitors
  - ❖ Theoretically, chemopreventive agents will require long-term use. Because NSAIDs show activity, yet have toxicities especially with long-term use, there is much interest in the new selective COX-2 inhibitors.
  - ❖ Basic research supports the lack of COX-2 expression in normal tissue, e.g., colonic mucosa, while demonstrating it is overexpressed in cancerous tumors, e.g., CRC.[9]
  - ❖ The COX-2 inhibitor celecoxib is FDA approved as adjunct to the usual care for patients with FAP, because it demonstrated a significant decrease in both the size and number of polyps.[10]
  - ❖ The success of celecoxib in FAP launched research interests in sporadic adenomas. There are three large multicenter trials underway looking at secondary prevention of sporadic adenomas after previous polypectomy. One sponsored is by the NCI; the other two are sponsored by the respective pharmaceutical companies. The results from the NCI trial, which is the most mature, might be available in a couple of years.
    1. Celecoxib 200 mg BID vs 400 mg BID vs placebo (NCI study)
    2. Celecoxib 400 mg daily vs placebo
    3. Rofecoxib 25 mg per day vs placebo
  - ❖ Little is known about the effects of aspirin, NSAIDs, or the COX-2 inhibitors on the development of polyps in HNPCC individuals. An

ongoing clinical trial is investigating the effect of celecoxib in individuals known to be carriers of HNPCC.

Prophylactic surgery

❖ In persons with severe dysplasia from ulcerative colitis, a colectomy should be considered.[11]

❖ In persons with FAP, a prophylactic colectomy with ileal pouch–anal anastomosis is recommended if there are 5 to 10 adenomatous polyps present or if polyps recur.[11]

❖ In persons with HNPCC, a subtotal or total colectomy may be considered, especially if there are 5 to 10 adenomatous polyps currently present or if polyps recur.[11]

❖ Women of HNPCC families, which have a high incidence of extracolonic tumors, should be presented with surgical options such as hysterectomy with an oophorectomy.

Possible Dietary Factors in Colorectal Cancer Prevention

❖ The development of CRC is probably influenced by dietary intake, while the role of diet in its prevention can be confusing, even controversial.

❖ Dietary fat
  ◆ Laboratory and observational studies have linked high fat intake to several health problems, including CRC. The mechanism between

dietary fat and CRC development is unclear. It has been suggested that it involves bile acids, a possible cancer promoter.[11] In addition, the fat in meats may contain carcinogens, which are released into the body when ingested.[12] The American (Western) diet is high in fat, making up 40% to 50% of the daily calories, and high in red meat.

❖ A new study provides the strongest correlation between a diet high in red meats and fast foods and an increased incidence of CRC. In addition, about half of the patients interviewed were found to have a mutated $p53$ gene in their colon tumors. The patients with this mutation were most likely to be the individuals who ate a high meat, fat, and sugar diet. Interestingly, people over the age of 65 also were more likely to have the mutation.[13] This study confirms the link between diet and cancer risk. The diet was associated with an increased risk regardless of the status of $p53$.[13] Even more important, it links diet to a specific cancer pathway demonstrating the importance of dietary modifications.[13]

❖ Overall, the results are very suggestive that dietary fat can increase colon cancer.[4,13] The American Cancer Society recommends a diet low in fat and processed and red meats, while high in fruits, vegetables, and whole grain foods.

❖ Dietary fiber

❖ Ingestion of fiber may alter colon carcinogenesis by a variety of means: increasing fecal bulk and transit time reducing exposure to carcinogens, and stimulation of bacterial fermentation and the subsequent production of short-chain fatty acids that may have anticarcinogenic effects, or decrease the process of bile acid production.

❖ The role of dietary fiber has been called into question. Previously it was felt to be protective, but recent data has been inconsistent.[14] Until additional research is completed, a high-fiber, low-fat diet is likely to be a benefit—if not for CRC prevention, then for cardiovascular disease.

❖ Dietary carcinogens

❖ Food additives, synthetic pesticides, etc., represent less than 1% of the carcinogens in our food. Most dietary carcinogens are produced by the plants themselves, e.g., toxins that protect the plant against insects, fungi, etc., or are by-products of food preparation.

❖ Only a few of the possible carcinogens produced by plant foods have been tested, making estimation of exposure difficult. Research is needed.

❖ Several known carcinogens are produced by food preparation and preservation methods.

   1. heterocyclic aromatic amines (HAAs) are formed during frying, grilling, and charring high-protein foods.

2. polycyclic aromatic hydrocarbons (PAHs) are formed during broiling and smoking foods.
3. *n*-nitroso compounds (NOCs) are formed when foods are salted, pickled, or cured with nitrate or nitrite.

❖ Research is needed to understand the complex interactions between all the dietary factors and their effect on the development of colorectal cancer.[15]

Relationship of Lifestyle Factors and Colorectal Cancer Prevention

❖ Physical activity and body weight

  ❖ A sedentary lifestyle and being overweight are both associated with an increased risk of CRC. These might not be independent factors but rather interrelated to each other and to the American obsession with convenience foods known to be high in calories and fat. Balancing energy expenditures with caloric intake through physical activity is a key to help protect against CRC. Physical activity stimulates the movement of stool through the colon, decreasing transit time, and reducing the exposure of the colonic mucosa to possible carcinogens.[16]

  ❖ The American Cancer Society (ACS) recommends a physically active lifestyle with 30–45 minutes of regular exercise 5+ days each week, maintenance of a healthy weight, and limiting the intake of high-fat animal source foods.[17]

❖ Hormone replacement therapy

* In postmenopausal women, several studies have shown that hormone replacement therapy (HRT) can reduce the incidence of CRC, but it also increases the risk of breast and uterine cancers.

* The U.S. Preventive Services Task Force recommends that all postmenopausal women should discuss the risks and benefits of HRT with their healthcare provider and balance that information with their own risks.[18]

❖ Alcohol consumption

* Epidemiologic studies show a direct relationship between beer consumption and rectal cancer

* Results are mixed about the association between colon cancer and alcohol consumption.

* The ACS recommends no more than two drinks per day for men and one drink per day for women.[17]

❖ Cigarette smoking

* Research has suggested an association between smoking and CRC. The link is primarily due to the fact that cigarettes contain thousands of chemicals including many known to be carcinogens and tumor promoters.

❖ Genetics is a factor in colon carcinogenesis, but it does not work in isolation. Environmental carcinogens and lifestyle factors may result in CRC regardless of an individual's genetic makeup, but patients with known genetic abnormalities may inherit a predisposition to abnormal cellular proliferation.[11] The recommended lifestyle modifications can be very beneficial in the prevention of many illness, e.g., cardiac disease if not also CRC.

Role of Clinical Trials in Colorectal Cancer Prevention

❖ Cancer clinical trials are research studies that answer key scientific questions in the areas of cancer treatment and prevention. Clinical trials are designed to have conclusions supported by data rather than theoretical reasoning. In addition, trials must follow all regulatory guidelines to provide safety to those participating.

❖ There are two types of prevention trials: those that investigate the effect of an intervention, e.g., dietary modification, or those that study the effect of an agent, e.g., medications or vitamins, on the incidence of cancer. Prevention trials are often placebo controlled, which would represent the usual behavior (control group of the trial). The studies may also be blinded to decrease any bias in efficacy or side-effect reporting.

❖ The participants in chemoprevention clinical trials are often individuals at high risk for either developing cancer for the first time or having their cancer recur. The number of participants involved in such research is often large (in the thousands), and the duration of therapy is commonly for 5 to 10 years. (It may take several years to impact carcinogenesis and then see an effect.)

❖ Participant adherence to the assigned intervention/agent is crucial to the overall success of the trial. For example, if a trial is comparing a COX-2 inhibitor versus placebo on the recurrence of CRC and some patients randomized to the placebo arm take either a NSAID agent or a COX-2 inhibitor for arthritis, the results will be skewed.

❖ Colorectal cancer prevention trials with various agents and interventions are ongoing both at the NCI and at cancer centers across the country. We have learned a lot about the impact of dietary fat, fiber, aspirin, NSAIDs, physical activity, as well as vitamins and minerals on the development of adenomas and colorectal tumors. We must continue this work to further our knowledge and impact CRC incidence in future generations.

"Real generosity towards the future lies in giving all to the present."

—Albert Camus (1913–1960), 1951

References

1. Loescher LJ. "Dynamics of Cancer Prevention." In Groenwald SL, Frogge MH, Goodman M, and Yarbro C, eds. *Cancer Nursing: Principles and Practice.* Boston, MA: Jones and Bartlett, 1997: 95.

2. Mayne ST, and Lippman SM. "Cancer Prevention: Chemopreventive Agents." In DeVita VT Jr, Frogge MH, Goodman M, and Yarbro C, eds. *Cancer: Principles & Practice of Oncology.* Philadelphia, PA: Lippincott-Raven, 1997: 585.

3. Loescher LJ. "Dynamics of Cancer Prevention." In Groenwald SL, Frogge MH, Goodman M, and Yarbro C, eds. *Cancer Nursing: Principles and Practice.* Boston, MA: Jones and Bartlett, 1997: 98.

4. Garay CA, Engstrom PF. "Chemoprevention of Colorectal Cancer: Dietary and Pharmacologic Approaches." *Oncology.* 1999; 13 (1): 89–98. Available at http://www.intouchlive.com/journals/oncology/o9901c .htm#Vitamins. Accessed July 12, 2002.

5. Clark LC, Combs GF Jr, Turnbull BW, *et al.* "Effects of Selenium Supplementation for Cancer Prevention in Patients with Carcinoma of the Skin." *JAMA.* 1997; 276: 1957–1963.

6. Bostick RM, Potter JD, McKenzie DR, *et al.* "Reduced Risk of Colon Cancer with High Intake of Vitamin E: The Iowa Women's Health Study." *Cancer Res.* 1993; 53: 4230–4237.

7. Ahnen DJ. Primary Preventive Measures for Colorectal Cancer. Presented at Ninth Annual Oncology Update for Primary Care, Omaha, NE, September 15, 2000.

8. Levin B. "COX-2 Inhibitors for Cancer Prevention and Therapy." ASCO Virtual Meeting. Available at

http://virtualmeeting.asco.org/vm2002/cancer.cfm. Accessed July 12, 2002.

9. Ahnen DJ. Primary Preventive Measures for Colorectal Cancer. Presented at Ninth Annual Oncology Update for Primary Care, Omaha, NE, September 15, 2000.

10. Steinbach G, Lynch PM, Phillips RK, *et al.* "The Effect of Celecoxib, a Cyclooxygenase-2 Inhibitor, in Familial Adenomatous Polyposis." *N Engl J Med.* 2000; 342: 1946–1952.

11. Goldberg RM. "Gastrointestinal Tract Cancers." In Casciato DA and Lowitz BB, eds. *Manual of Clinical Oncology*, 4th ed. Philadelphia, PA: Lippincott Williams & Wilkins, 2000: 182–194.

12. Cohen AM, Minsky BD, and Schilsky RL. "Cancer of the Colon." In DeVita VT Jr, Rosenberg SA, and Hellman S, eds. *Cancer: Principles & Practice of Oncology.* Philadelphia, PA: Lippincott-Raven, 1997: 1146.

13. American Cancer Society. "Pass on the Burgers and Fries, and Lower the Risk for Colon Cancer." June 16, 2002. Available at www.cancer.org/eprise/main/docroot/cri/cri-0. Accessed June 28, 2002.

14. Ellenhorn JDI, Coia LR, Alberts SR, and Hoff PM. "Colorectal and Anal Cancers." In Pazdur R, Coia LR, Hoskins HJ, and Wagman LD, eds. *Cancer Management: A Multidisciplinary Approach*, 6th ed. Melville, NY: PRR, Inc, 2002: 295–318.

15. Greenwald P. "Cancer Prevention: Dietary Carcinogens." In DeVita VT Jr, Rosenberg SA, and Hellman S, eds. *Cancer: Principles & Practice of Oncology.* Philadelphia, PA: Lippincott-Raven, 1997: 579–583.

16. Christiansen K. "Prevention Strategies and the Diet Connection." In Berg, D., ed. *Contemporary Issues in Colorectal Cancer: A Nursing Perspective.* Boston, MA: Jones and Bartlett Publishers, 2001: 35–52.

17. American Cancer Society. The Complete Guide—Nutrition and Physical Activity. February 21, 2002. Available at http://www.cancer.org/eprise/main/doc-root/PED/content/PED-3-2X-Diet-and-Activity-Factors-That-Affect-Risks?sitearea=PED. Accessed June 28, 2002.

18. University of Nebraska Medical College (UNMC). UNMC Initiates Local Research Study on Hormone Replacement Therapy. Available at www.unmc.edu/News/hrt/htm. Accessed June 28, 2002.

PART II

Disease Assessment

5

Natural History of Cancers of the Colon and Rectum: Pathophysiology and Disease Manifestations

Introduction

We now have a clearer understanding of the natural history and biologic features of colorectal cancer (CRC). We have a better insight into the genetic influences as well. What genetic changes occur and when, as well as biologic features, are the basis for new areas of prevention and therapeutic research. Understanding the disease manifestations and the means of progression can provide the background for clinical interventions, which can make a difference for people suffering from CRC.

Carcinogenesis

❖ Under normal conditions the division, proliferation, and differentiation of colonic epithelial cells is strictly balanced.

❖ Any disruption in this balance can result in an adenomatous formation. If allowed to grow unchecked, and if there are additional influences, the adenoma can grow into an invasive tumor.

❖ CRC is attributable to multiple forces (an accumulation of genetic mutations that result from a series of events occurring through many different pathways) that drive the transformation (an imbalance between cellular proliferation and death) of colorectal mucous to CRC.[3]

❖ Proto-oncogenes encode for proteins, which regulate cell proliferation. When there is a mutation in the proto-oncogene, it is "activated" and is called an oncogene.

❖ Tumor-suppressor genes are those that normally suppress cell proliferation. When there is a mutation, an inactivation or deletion, control of proliferation is lost and growth goes unchecked.

❖ Growth abnormalities of tumor cells result from both too little of the tumor-suppressor action and too much of the oncogene-accelerator action.

❖ Loss of apoptosis (programmed cell death) signals may be a critical mutational event in carcinogenesis.[1,2]

❖ Known genetic changes in colorectal cancer
  ❖ Tumor suppressor genes
    1. Adenomatous polyposis coli (APC) gene—considered one of the initial mutations,

which leads to hyperproliferation of the epithelial tissue lining the colon

2. Deleted in colon cancer (DCC) gene—found in 80% of CRC, loss leads to a benign adenoma
3. *p53*—found in 75% of CRC tumors, felt to increase the risk of CRC, contributes to inappropriate progression through the cell cycle even after DNA damage, increased genetic instability, and decreased apoptosis[1,2]

❖ Oncogenes

1. C-Myc gene amplification—associated with progression from small to large adenoma and ultimately cancer
2. Ras oncogenes, e.g., K-Ras1—found in 50% of all carcinomas and larger adenomas; thought to be responsible for the change from adenoma to adenocarcinoma[3]

❖ Mismatch repair genes

1. *h*MSH2, *h*MLH1, *h*PMS1, *h*PMS2, *h*MSH3, and *h*MSH6—add to the instability of the cell

❖ Miscellaneous mutations

1. Allele deletion on chromosomes 5, 17, and 18 add to the cells' ability to progress from normal to malignant colonic mucosa.[3]

❖ One probable schema for CRC carcinogenesis is outlined in Figure 5-1.

FIGURE 5–1

A conceptual genetic model for the development of colorectal cancer, illustrating multistep carcinogenesis

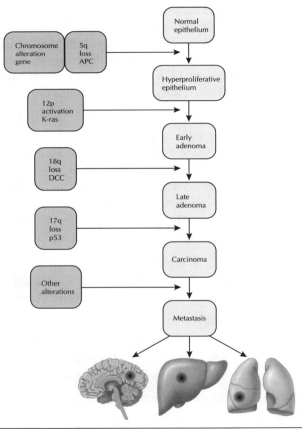

Source: Griffin-Sobel, JP. "Cellular Characteristics, Pathophysiology, and Disease Manifestations of Colorectal Cancer." In Berg, D, ed. *Contemporary Issues in Colorectal Cancer: A Nursing Perspective.* Boston, MA: Jones and Bartlett Publishers, 2001: 53–64

Disease Manifestations

❖ Figure 5-2 and 5-3: Anatomy of the colon and rectum[4]

❖ Figure 5-4 outlines the layers of the colon.[4]

❖ Cellular division takes place in the crypts of Lieberkuhn in the mucosal layer. As new cells are produced, they mature, migrate up and out of the crypt, and are shed into the lumen. Damage to the crypts can result in errors in cell division and the formation of adenomas (polyps).

FIGURE 5-2
Anatomy of the colon

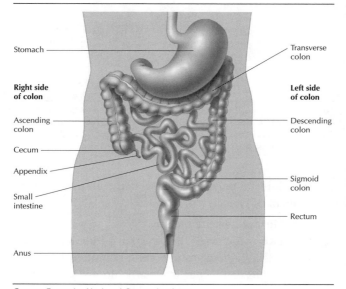

Source: From the National Cancer Institute.

FIGURE 5-3
Anatomy of the rectum

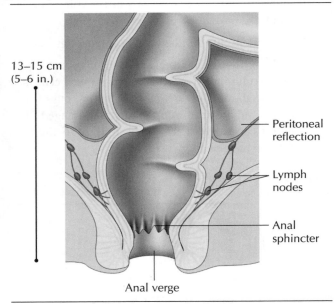

13–15 cm
(5–6 in.)

Peritoneal
reflection

Lymph
nodes

Anal
sphincter

Anal verge

Source: Griffin-Sobel, JP. "Cellular Characteristics, Pathophysiology, and Disease Manifestations of Colorectal Cancer." In Berg, D, ed. *Contemporary Issues in Colorectal Cancer: A Nursing Perspective.* Boston, MA: Jones and Bartlett Publishers, 2001: 53–64

❖ Colorectal polyps are associated with the development of cancer.
  ❖ Most polyps are benign.
  ❖ Two major types: pedunculated (tubular) and sessile (villous) as pictured in Figure 5-5
  ❖ Polyps can be detected early, do not penetrate the submucosa for several years, but once they

FIGURE 5-4
Layers of the colon noting tumor penetration

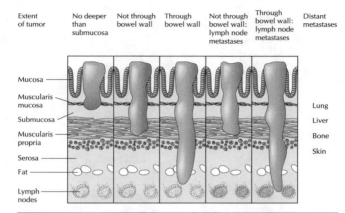

Source: Griffin-Sobel, JP. "Cellular Characteristics, Pathophysiology, and Disease Manifestations of Colorectal Cancer." In Berg, D, ed. *Contemporary Issues in Colorectal Cancer: A Nursing Perspective.* Boston, MA: Jones and Bartlett Publishers, 2001: 53–64

reach the muscularis, they are likely to become malignant and invasive.[1,5]

- ❖ Histologic types of CRC
  - ❖ Adenocarcinoma is most common type, accounting for 98% of tumors.[3,6]
  - ❖ Mucinous carcinomas: produce large amounts of extracellular mucous; tend to spread within the peritoneum; account for 10% of tumors; are more common in younger patients

FIGURE 5-5
Neoplastic polyps: Pedunculated (stalk) and sessile

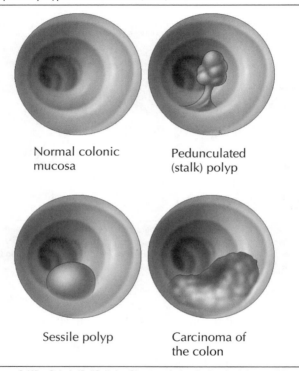

Normal colonic
mucosa

Pedunculated
(stalk) polyp

Sessile polyp

Carcinoma of
the colon

Source: Griffin-Sobel, JP. "Cellular Characteristics, Pathophysiology, and Disease Manifestations of Colorectal Cancer." In Berg, D, ed. *Contemporary Issues in Colorectal Cancer: A Nursing Perspective*. Boston, MA: Jones and Bartlett Publishers, 2001: 53–64

* Signet-ring cell carcinomas: account for 1% of tumors; are difficult to detect
* Squamous cell, small cell, carcinoids, and adenosquamous tumors are infrequent.
* Lymphomas, sarcomas, and melanomas are rare.

* Cancer can occur anywhere in the colon.[7]

  * Common incidences
    1. 14% arise in the rectum.
    2. 35% arise in the sigmoid colon.
    3. 7% arise in the descending colon.
    4. 10% occur in the transverse colon.
    5. 12% occur in the ascending colon.
    6. 22% occur in the cecum.

  * Incidence is shifting to the proximal from the distal segments of the colon.[1]

  * Lesion characteristics within the different colonic segments[1,8]

    1. Tumors in ascending colon

       a. Cauliflower-like fungating masses that become ulcerative and necrotic
       b. Usually well differentiated, are more genetically stable, and carry a better prognosis[1,3,8]

    2. Tumors in descending and sigmoid colon

       a. Usually ulcerative tumors that tend to infiltrate the bowel wall
       b. Show more genetic instability and carry a poorer prognosis[1,3,8]

3. Rectosigmoid tumors

a. Usually are villous, frondlike tumors

❖ At diagnosis, 25% of colon cancers have spread through the bowel wall, while 50% to 70% of rectal cancers have spread through the wall.[6]

❖ Cancer metastasis

❖ Figure 5-6 shows the metastatic cascade.

❖ Metastasis is a complex process with a number of essential steps.

1. Progressive proliferation[1]

a. Local invasion by circumferential growth of enlarging cancer mass can invade surrounding tissues and lymphatics directly resulting in visceral and lymphatic metastasis. Longitudinal spread is usually not extensive averaging less than 1–2 cm from the tumor.

2. Development of a vasculature (angiogenesis)[1,5]

a. Substances that promote vascularization: vascular endothelial growth factor (VEGF); epideral growth factor (EGF); interleukin-8 (IL-8); granulocyte colony-stimulating factor (G-CSF); and tumor necrosis factor-alfa (TNF-a)

b. Substances that inhibit vascularization: tumor growth factor beta-1 (TGF-B1), alfa-interferon, angiostatin, endostatin, and platelet factor[9]

FIGURE 5-6

The metastatic cascade. The multistep cascade begins when genetic events facilitate primary tumor formation. Angiogenesis (vascularization) increases proliferation of the growing tumor. Preceding invasion, there is a decrease in cell-cell contact and adherence to and invasion of the endothelial basement membrane. Once tumor cells have entered the lymphatic system or circulation, they are transported to distant sites. If the tumor cells are successful at evading the immune system, they eventually will arrest in a capillary bed of a distant organ. Establishment of a secondary site will follow once the tumor cells invade the endothelial barrier to gain entrance to the underlying organ tissue bed.

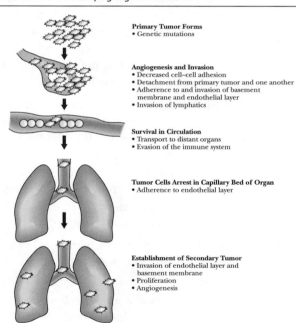

Primary Tumor Forms
• Genetic mutations

Angiogenesis and Invasion
• Decreased cell–cell adhesion
• Detachment from primary tumor and one another
• Adherence to and invasion of basement membrane and endothelial layer
• Invasion of lymphatics

Survival in Circulation
• Transport to distant organs
• Evasion of the immune system

Tumor Cells Arrest in Capillary Bed of Organ
• Adherence to endothelial layer

Establishment of Secondary Tumor
• Invasion of endothelial layer and basement membrane
• Proliferation
• Angiogenesis

Source: Gribbon J, Loescher LJ. "Biology of Cancer." In Yarbro CH, Frogge MH, Goodman M. *et al. Cancer Nursing: Principles and Practice*, 5th ed. Sudbury, MA: Jones and Bartlett, 2000, 31. With permission.

   3. Penetration through normal blood vessels[1,5]

      a. Matrix-degrading enzymes support the penetration through the vessel wall.[1]

      b. Cancer cells invade blood vessels and can be transported by the circulatory system to distant sites. Cells entering the circulation are rapidly destroyed by immune surveillance unless they form into a mass for protection. The formation of fibrin deposits and platelet aggregation as a tumor protector is well documented.[5]

      c. The increased coagulability seen in cancer patients may be related to high levels of thromboplastin and the production of procoagulants by some tumors.[1,5]

 ❖ The therapeutic potential to intervene in these processes is being widely studied. For example, matrix metalloproteinases (MMP) inhibitors may prevent cells from traveling via the circulation; antiangiogenesis agents may prevent the development of new blood vessels needed to support the tumor.

 ❖ Common sites of metastases

   1. Colon: liver, lymph nodes, peritoneal cavity, lungs, bones, and adrenals. Brain metastasis is rare.

      a. The venous system of the colon and proximal rectum drain into the portal system, resulting in the liver being the most frequent site of metastasis.[9]

    b. At diagnosis, approximately 37% of colon tumors have already metastasized to the regional lymph nodes.[10]

  2. Rectum: lymph nodes, lung, liver, intra-abdominal and -peritoneal spread

    a. The inferior vena cava is the primary drainage from the rectal area so pulmonary metastasis is common.

    b. At diagnosis 50% to 60% of rectal tumors have already metastasized to regional lymph nodes.[6]

    c. Intraperitoneal seeding and carcinomatosis are more common with rectal tumors than colon tumors.[1]

❖ Patterns of disease failure[6]

  ❖ The patterns of disease failure are different between colon and rectal cancer.

    1. Locoregional failure is three times more common with rectal cancer.[3]

    2. Distant failure is common with colon cancer.

  ❖ These differences dictate treatment strategies.

References

1. DeVita V, Hellman S, and Rosenberg S. *Cancer: Principles and Practices of Oncology*, 6th ed. Philadelphia, PA: Lippincott-Raven, 2001.

2. Glaser E, and Grogan L. Molecular genetics of GI malignancies. *Semin Oncol Nurs.* 1999; 15(1): 3–10.

3. Goldberg RM. Gastrointestinal Tract Cancers. In Casciato DA, and Lowitz BB, eds. *Manual of Clinical Oncology*, 4th ed. Philadelphia, PA: Lippincott Williams & Wilkins, 2000: 182–194.

4. Griffin-Sobel, JP. Cellular Characteristics, Pathophysiology, and Disease Manifestations of Colorectal Cancer. In Berg, D, ed. *Contemporary Issues in Colorectal Cancer: A Nursing Perspective*. Boston, MA: Jones and Bartlett Publishers, 2001: 53–64.

5. McCance K, and Huether S. *Pathophysiology: The Biologic Basis for Disease in Adults and Children*, 3rd ed. St. Louis, MO: Mosby, 1998.

6. Ellenhorn JDI, Coia LR, Alberts SR, and Hoff PM. Colorectal and anal cancers. In Pazdur R, Coia LR, Hoskins HJ, and Wagman LD, eds. *Cancer Management: A Multidisciplinary Approach*, 6th ed. Melville, NY: PRR, Inc, 2002: 295–318.

7. MayoClinic.com. Colorectal cancer. February 4, 2002. Available at http://www.mayoclinic.com/findinformation/diseasesandconditions/invoke.cfm?id=DS00035. Accessed July 12, 2002.

8. Curtas S. Diagnosing GI malignancies. *Semin Oncol Nurs*. 1999; 15(1): 10–16.

9. Macdonald JS. Cancer chemotherapy and the liver. *Clin Liver Dis*. 1998; 2(3): 631–642.

10. Jemal A, Thomas A, Murray T, and Thun M. Cancer statistics, 2002. *CA Cancer J Clin*. 2002; 52(1): 23–47.

6

Assessment, Diagnosis, and Staging

Introduction

Clinical presentation, signs and symptoms, assessment, diagnosis, and staging of the patient with colon or rectal cancer (CRC) are important in the overall clinical care. Therapeutic options and survival depend on one very key factor—the extent of disease at the time of diagnosis.

Clinical Presentation

❖ CRC develops from a polyp on the mucosal lining that was not found or removed. The polyp became malignant and continued to grow, often spreading through some or all of the bowel wall. Once outside the bowel wall, the malignant cells invade nearby organs, lymph nodes, and blood vessels, and spread to distant sites.

❖ Approximately 56% of tumors develop in the left colon (i.e., descending, sigmoid, and rectal areas).[1]

❖ Approximately 34% develop in the right colon (i.e., cecum and ascending colon).[1]

❖ Approximately 10% develop in the transverse colon.[1]

❖ CRC spreads outward through the layers of the colon and inward decreasing the size of the lumen.

❖ The location of the tumor within a specific segment of the colon or rectum helps dictate the direction and sites of metastasis.

  ❖ Tumors in the ascending or descending colon spread to the retroperitoneal tissue, kidney, ureter, or pancreas.
  ❖ The colon and proximal rectum drain into the portal system, thereby tumors frequently spread to the liver.
  ❖ The distal rectum passes directly into the inferior vena cava, as a result tumors commonly spread to the lung.[2] Approximately 10% of patients with rectal carcinoma will have lung metastasis at diagnosis.[3]
  ❖ Other sites of metastatic disease that could lead to clinical presentation are lymph nodes, bone, and peritoneum. Metastasis to the brain is rare.[4]

CRC Signs and Symptoms

❖ CRC is often asymptomatic until the tumor is well advanced, thereby blocking the flow of stool, developing into a palpable mass, or causing organ dysfunction secondary to metastasis.

❖ The signs and symptoms frequently associated with CRC are:

- ❖ Bright red blood with bowel movements
- ❖ Stools that are tarry black or have mucus
- ❖ Change in bowel habits (e.g., constipation, diarrhea, or alternation between the two, lasting more than a few days)
- ❖ Change in size, shape, or color of the stool (e.g., ribbon-like or narrower stools)
- ❖ Difficulty having a bowel movement
- ❖ Feeling of incomplete stooling (tenesmus)
- ❖ Stomach or abdominal discomfort, cramping, or pain, colicky or gnawing in nature
- ❖ Abdominal fullness, bloating, or distention
- ❖ Unusual and/or continuing fatigue
- ❖ Unexplained weight loss or gain
- ❖ Jaundice

❖ When present, symptoms are often minor, ignored, or misinterpreted as being caused by other conditions.

- ❖ Bright red bleeding is common with hemorrhoids.
- ❖ Abdominal cramping, pain, gas and changes in bowel habits are often confused with irritable bowel syndrome, diverticular disease, ischemic colitis, inflammatory bowel disease, infectious colitis, hemorrhoids, and intolerance to specific foods.

❖ Signs and symptoms of CRC can vary based on the location of the tumor within the colon (i.e., right-sided tumors vs. left-sided tumors) (Figure 6-1).

FIGURE 6–1
Signs and symptoms of colorectal cancer

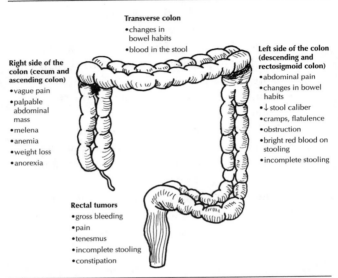

Transverse colon
- changes in bowel habits
- blood in the stool

Right side of the colon (cecum and ascending colon)
- vague pain
- palpable abdominal mass
- melena
- anemia
- weight loss
- anorexia

Left side of the colon (descending and rectosigmoid colon)
- abdominal pain
- changes in bowel habits
- ↓ stool caliber
- cramps, flatulence
- obstruction
- bright red blood on stooling
- incomplete stooling

Rectal tumors
- gross bleeding
- pain
- tenesmus
- incomplete stooling
- constipation

Source: Sweed MR, Meropol NJ. "Assessment, Diagnosis, and Staging." In Berg, D. ed. *Contemporary Issues in Colorectal Cancer: A Nursing Perspective.* Boston, MA: Jones and Bartlett Publishers, 2001: 65–79. Reprinted with permission.

❖ The colon is a flexible tube. The materials that pass through it start as liquid in the right colon and end as a solid material once it reaches the rectum.

❖ Tumors in the right colon often exhibit different symptoms and at a later stage than tumors in the left colon.

❖ Metastases to the liver may present with hepatomegally and/or a knobby, irregular surface.

❖ Once suspected, a complete work-up is initiated to rule out or detect a primary tumor or a site of metastasis.

Making the Initial Diagnosis

❖ History (Table 6-1 Important Recommended Questions)[5]

  ❖ Prior surgical and medical history

    1. Social history, i.e., smoking and alcohol consumption
    2. Individual and family history, especially noted risk factors for CRC
    3. Details about any presenting signs and symptoms, remembering they are often vague

  ❖ Information can focus the physical examination, guide the imaging tests, and help determine the differential diagnoses.

❖ Complete physical examination

  ❖ Survey lymph nodes, breast, abdomen, and rectum assessing for primary lesions or sites of metastasis

  ❖ Abdominal assessment: signs of temporal or masseter wasting (indicative of severe weight loss), abdominal distention (suggestive of ascites), palpable masses, areas of tenderness, signs of bowel perforation, abdominal auscultation looking for hypermotility

TABLE 6-1
The History: Questions to Ask

❖ How old are you?

❖ How would you describe your ethnic background or race?

❖ Is there a personal or family history of polyps?

❖ Do you have a history of ulcerative colitis, diverticulitis, or Crohn's disease?

❖ Have you ever been told you have hemorrhoids or anal fissures?

❖ Have you ever had blood in your stools?

❖ Have you ever had a problem emptying your bowels?

❖ Is there a family history of colon or rectal cancer? (Include extended family)

❖ Is there a personal or family history of endometrial, ovarian, gastric, or urinary tract malignancy?

❖ How old was the person at the time of the cancer diagnosis?

❖ Has there been a change in your bowel habits?

❖ Do you smoke or have you smoked cigarettes, cigars, etc.?

❖ How would you describe your intake of alcohol?

Source: Sweed MR, and Meropol NJ. "Assessment, Diagnosis, and Staging." In Berg, D. ed. *Contemporary Issues in Colorectal Cancer: A Nursing Perspective.* Boston, MA: Jones and Bartlett Publishers, 2001: 65–79. Reprinted with permission.

(indicative of partial bowel obstruction), or weak or absent bowel sounds (suggestive of complete bowel obstruction). Palpable masses are more common with tumors located in the right colon. Acute perforation may present with pain, fever, and a palpable mass. Chronic perforation with fistula formation into the bladder, from sigmoid tumors, can present as recurrent urinary tract infections and gross hematuria. Right flank, posterior chest, or upper quadrant pain, scleral icterus, and jaundice may represent liver metastasis.

❖ Pelvic examination: Rectal assessment by digital rectal examination to assess for masses, including prostate examination in men.[2] Women with complaints of pelvic pain (potentially from ovarian or cul-de-sac metastases) should undergo a pelvic examination.

❖ A neurologic exam may uncover suspicious metastatic brain disease or ensuing spinal cord compression.

❖ Other systemic physical findings may aid in the diagnosis of CRC.

1. Metastasis at the umbilicus metastases (Sister Joseph nodules)
2. Peutz-Jeghers syndrome is associated with gastrointestinal (GI) tract polyposis.[6,7]
3. Sebaceous skin tumors may be a sign of Muir-Torre syndrome (hereditary colon cancer).
4. Paraneoplastic syndromes:
   a. Acanthosis nigricans (symmetric, hyper-pigmented, velvety skin thickening usually at the neck, axillae, antecubital, popliteal fossae, periumbilical area, and groin)
   b. Dermatomyositis (dermatitis and inflammation of the muscles)

      c. Hypercalcemia occurs due a parathyroid hormone (PTH)-like activity; it is very common in people with cancer. Signs and symptoms: lethargy, confusion, dehydration, constipation, abdominal pain, nausea, and vomiting

      d. Hypercoagulability (i.e., superficial or deep vein thrombosis with or without pulmonary embolism)[8]

❖ Laboratory tests

  ❖ Complete blood count (CBC), serum chemistries, including liver and renal function, and coagulation assays are initially ordered.

    1. Anemia often triggers investigation with a colonoscopy, as most individuals, except menstruating females, are not usually anemic.

    2. Liver function tests, such as alkaline phosphatase and gamma-glutamyl-transpeptidase (GGT), offer important information about the possibility of liver and bone metastases respectively.[8,9]

    3. Hypercoagulability conditions are commonly seen with CRC.[8,9]

  ❖ Investigational tests: Molecular analysis of stool searching for specific DNA mutations, e.g., mutations in the *RAS* gene[10,11]

❖ Colonic examination

  ❖ Goal: determine the primary site of disease

❖ Options:

1. Endoscopic procedures—sigmoidoscopy and colonoscopy
2. Radiographic procedure—double contrast barium enema; if positive an endoscopic procedure will be necessary to biopsy lesions.
3. Test is selected based on the suspected location of the lesion and patient issues.
4. Limitations of the different colonic examinations were illustrated in Chapter 3.
5. Biopsy of suspicious lesions is mandatory to make a diagnosis.

❖ Investigational tests:

1. Computerized tomography (CT) colonography (also called virtual colonoscopy, virtual endoscopy, 3D-endoscopy, and CT colography) is a newer technique combining CT data and digital images; if positive, an endoscopic procedure will be necessary to biopsy lesions.
2. Immunoscintigraphy—Oncoscint and CEA-scan are newer diagnostic scans used primarily to detect recurrent disease.

Work Up After Confirming the Cancer Diagnosis

❖ Goal: determine all the site(s) and clinical stage of disease

❖ Preoperative testing to assess for extracolonic disease (staging purposes)

❖ Chest x-ray

- ❖ CT scans of the abdomen, pelvis, and chest (unless a chest x-ray performed)
- ❖ Other imaging studies: magnetic resonance, positron emission tomography scans, transrectal ultrasound
- ❖ Blood tests: CBC and serum chemistry, if not done prediagnosis, and urinalysis. Serum carcinoembryonic antigen (CEA) and CA-19-9

   1. CEA is a tumor-associated marker not a tumor-specific marker and is elevated in cancers and conditions other than colorectal cancer. Normal CEA levels <2.5 ng/mL for nonsmokers and <5.0 ng/mL for smokers; thus, overexpression is suspicious for cancer.[12] Preoperative CEA assessment is crucial because elevated levels correlate with stage and outcome; postoperatively levels return to normal within 4 to 6 weeks.[13] The American Society of Clinical Oncology (ASCO) recommends the use of CEA to help detect recurrence or progression (new elevations after normalization are often representative of disease), and to determine the response to or failure of treatment for metastatic disease.[14]

   2. Lipid-associated sialic acid (LASA), CA 19-9, DNA ploidy, *p*53, and *ras* are experimental tumor markers and are not recommended for use in therapeutic decisions, but rather may be performed in the context of a clinical trial.[14]

- ❖ Transrectal ultrasound

1. Valuable for staging of rectal tumors as treatment decisions are made, preoperative versus postoperative adjuvant therapy, based on the clinical staging with ultrasound
2. Highly accurate (95%) at defining the depth of penetration[4,15]
3. Approximately 62% of the time enlarged lymph nodes are diagnosed, again affecting treatment decisions.[15]

❖ CT scanning is useful in detecting tumors in the chest, abdomen, or pelvis, particularly pulmonary and hepatic metastases. Sensitivity is increased with intravenous contrast. Helical (spiral) CT provides greater detail and can be even more useful in evaluating metastatic disease.[16]

❖ A bone scan can be helpful in the setting of persistent bone pain, but it is not required for everyone.[7]

❖ Magnetic resonance imaging (MRI)

1. Useful in detecting recurrent disease, especially questionable abnormalities visualized in the liver by CT, and detecting pelvic side-wall or sacral involvement. It is also used for preoperative staging.[17]

❖ Positron emission tomography (PET)

1. PET scanning utilizes the increased rate of glycolysis in tumor cells to detect malignancy. PET scanning is approved by many third-party payers to detect CRC recurrence.

It is often used to detect liver or lung metastasis in the context of elevated CEA levels and no evidence of disease.[18] The role of PET scanning in diabetic patients, who do not have optimal glycemic control, is limited.

❖ Recommended preparations for both endoscopic procedures and imaging tests are noted in Table 6-2.

Patterns of Disease Failure[19]

❖ Locoregional failure is common with rectal cancer.

❖ Distant failure is common with colon cancer.

Pathology

❖ Therapeutic planning and determination of prognosis require a careful tissue (pathologic) diagnosis.

  ❖ The tissue may be obtained from either a primary or metastatic site.

  ❖ Needle aspirates for cytologic analysis are often adequate for diagnosis of metastatic disease.[5]

❖ Pathologic evaluation includes histopathologic type (e.g., adenocarcinoma, signet ring cell carcinoma, squamous carcinoma, small cell carcinoma, undifferentiated carcinoma) and grade (well-, moderately, poorly, or undifferentiated). The most common histopathologic type is adenocarcinoma while most tumors are moderately differentiated.

❖ Additional pathologic information that may be useful includes ploidy (number of chromosomes),

TABLE 6–2
Imaging, Endoscopy, and Preparation

Study	Preparation	Aftercare
Barium Enema	Day before start clear liquids only 5 P.M. night before ⟹ 12oz Magnesium citrate 6 P.M. night before ⟹ 4 Dulcolax tablets No eating/drinking/smoking day of test Rectal suppository day of test	Drink at least 32 oz liquids within 24 hours after exam. Recommend laxative to facilitate passage of barium.
Cat Scan (abdominal & pelvis)	No eating, drinking or smoking for 3 hours before test. May drink 24 oz of contrast 1 hr prior to exam Frequently IV iodine contrast Need steroid pre-med for iodine allergy	If IV contrast injected, recommend 32 oz of fluid over next 24 hours.
Bone Scan	IV injection of a chemical compound, labeled with a small amt of radioactive material	none

(continued)

TABLE 6-2
Imaging, Endoscopy, and Preparation (continued)

Study	Preparation	Aftercare
MRI	For endorectal & pelvis studies: NPO 1 hr before the study. Will get glucagon injection to slow bowel to lessen motion on pictures. Because of strong magnetic field, need to check the following: pacemakers, ear implants, aneurysm clips, other metal, shrapnel, eye exposure to metal shavings, permanent make-up (contains lead). Pt must weigh <300 lbs.	No eating of solid foods for 3 hours if glucagons used. May only drink liquids immediately after glucagon or cramping will occur.
PET Scan	Nothing to eat/drink 4 hrs before except H_2O. Blood sugar must be <140mg/ml in order to be accurate. IV injection of radioactively labeled glucose. Entire procedure lasts 2–3 hrs	none
Rectal Ultrasound	6 P.M. night before ⇒ 1 bottle magnesium citrate Nothing to eat/drink after midnight Take 2 Fleet enemas 30 minutes apart 90 minutes before leaving home	

(continued)

TABLE 6-2
Imaging, Endoscopy, and Preparation (continued)

Study	Preparation	Aftercare
Sigmoidoscopy	Same as rectal ultrasound	
	Stop any medications containing aspirin, nonsteriodal anti-inflammatory drugs, anticoagulants, Persantine, Ticlid, Plavix for 7 days prior to testing	
Colonoscopy	Clear liquids start breakfast the day before. Evening before add 1 and ½ oz Fleet Phospho Soda to 4 oz of any clear liquid. Follow with another 8 oz. Drink a total of 3 more 8 oz glasses of clears before bedtime	Need to have someone to drive patient home after conscious sedation.
	Day of scope: 1 and ½ fluid oz Phospho-Soda to 4 oz of clear liquid. Follow with 8 oz liquid	
	IV conscious sedation is given.	
	Stop any meds containing aspirin, nonsteriodal anti-inflammatory drugs, anticoagulants, Persatine, Ticlid, Plavix for 7 days prior	

Source: Sweed MR, and Meropol NJ. "Assessment, Diagnosis, and Staging." In Berg, D. ed. *Contemporary Issues in Colorectal Cancer: A Nursing Perspective.* Boston, MA: Jones and Bartlett Publishers, 2001: 65–79. Reprinted with permission.

S-phrase fraction (indicative of rate of cellular proliferation), monoclonal antibody staining of tissue for anti-CEA and anti-TAG-72, cellular enzymes (thymidine phosphorylase and thymidylate synthase that may predict response to 5-fluorouracil therapy), and genetic abnormalities.

Staging

❖ Accurate staging is critical to establishing both therapeutic strategies and prognosis.

❖ Staging of CRC is based on depth of tumor penetration through the bowel wall, presence or absence of regional lymph node involvement, and presence or absence of distant metastases. In addition, the number of positive lymph nodes is considered.

❖ In contrast to many other cancers, tumor size is not included in CRC staging.

❖ Table 6-3 outlines the American Joint Commission on Cancer (AJCC) Tumor-Node-Metastasis (TNM) system.[21] The TNM system is the recommended system.[4]

❖ Staging at diagnosis and implications for long-term outcomes

 ❖ Early diagnosis correlates with a more favorable long-term outcome.

  1. Localized disease, that which is confined within the layers of the bowel wall, has a 90%

TABLE 6-3
TNM Classification and Staging of Colon and Rectal Cancer

Stage	Tumor (N)	Nodes (N)	Metastasis (M)
		Characteristics	
Stage 0	Carcinoma in situ	No regional lymph node involvement	No distant metastases
Stage I T1 N0 M0 T2 N0 M0	Tumor invades submucosa or muscularis propria	No regional lymph node involvement	No distant metastases
Stage II A T3 N0 M0	Tumor invades into the subserosa, or into nonperitonealized pericolic or perirectal tissue	No regional lymph node involvement	No distant metastases
B T4 N0 M0	Tumor directly (macroscopically) invades other organs (including other segments of the colorectum) or structures, and/or perforates visceral peritoneum. *	No regional lymph node involvement	No distant metastases
Stage III A T1-2 N1 M0	Invades submucosa or muscularis propria	Metastasis in 1 to 3 regional lymph nodes	No distant metastasis

(continued)

TABLE 6-3
TNM Classification and Staging of Colon and Rectal Cancer (continued)

Stage	Tumor (N)	Nodes (N)	Metastasis (M)
		Characteristics	
B T3-4 N1 M0	Invades into subserosa, or into nonperitonealized pericolic or perirectal tissue, or invades into other organs or structures, and/or perforates visceral peritoneum.*	Metastasis in 1 to 3 regional lymph nodes	No distant metastasis
C Any T N2 M0	Any tumor depth or involvement	Metastasis in 4+ regional lymph nodes	No distant metastasis
Stage IV Any T Any N M0	Any tumor depth or involvement	Any number of lymph nodes involved	Any distant metastasis

Source: Greene FL, Page DL, Fleming ID, Fritz AG, Balch CM, Haller DG, and Morrow M, eds. *American Joint Committee on Cancer Cancer Staging Manual*, 6th ed. *Colorectal Cancer*. New York, NY: Springer. 2002: 113–123.

5-year survival.[1] Unfortunately, only about 37% of people are diagnosed this early.[1]

2. Regional disease, that which has spread outside the bowel wall into nearby organs or lymph nodes, has a 66% 5-year survival. Again unfortunately, only about 37% of people are diagnosed with regional CRC.[1]

3. Metastatic disease, that which has spread not only outside the bowel wall but has spread to distant sites, has a 9% 5-year survival. Twenty-five percent of people are diagnosed with metastatic disease.[1]

Predictive Markers and Prognosis

❖ Table 6-4 outlines predictive markers and their association with prognosis.

❖ Conflicting data exist with regard to age at diagnosis, elevated CEA (>5mg/mL), gender, presence and duration of symptoms, site of disease, perineural invasion, ploidy status, and S-phase fraction and prognosis-disease recurrence or survival.[4,19]

The Role of the Nurse

❖ Know the signs and symptoms of CRC

❖ Educate patients, families, and friends about the warning signs of this disease and promote screening and early detection

TABLE 6-4
Predictive Markers and Prognosis.[4,19,20]

Poor Prognosis	Better Prognosis
Poorly differentiated grade	Well and moderated differentiated grade
Lymphatic or vascular invasion	Microsatellite instability (MSI)
*p*53 mutations	Aggressive lymph node dissection[20]
Absent deleted in colon cancer (DCC) gene	Early stage disease, i.e., stage I and II
High thymidylate synthase (TS) expression[19]	Low thymidylate syntase (TS) expression[19]
K-*ras* mutations	
Thymidine phosphorylase expression	
Metastases to regional lymph nodes	
Allele loss of chromosome18q	
Obstruction or perforation at presentation	

❧ Encourage individuals with possible signs of CRC to seek medical evaluation

❧ Assist individuals through the diagnostic work-up by providing information and support

References

1. MayoClinic.com. "Colorectal Cancer." February 4, 2002. Available at http://www.mayoclinic.com/find-information/diseasesandconditions/invoke.cfm?id=DS0 0035. Accessed July 12, 2002.

2. Cohen AM, Minsky BD, and Schilsky RL. "Cancer of the Colon." In DeVita V, Hellman S, and Rosenberg S, eds. *Cancer: Principles and Practice of Oncology*, 5th ed. Philadelphia, PA: Lippincott-Raven, 1997: 1144–1187.

3. Vignati PV, and Roberts PL. "Preoperative Evaluation and Postoperative Surveillance for Patients with Colorectal Cancer." *Surg Clin North Am.* 1993; 73: 67–84.

4. Goldberg RM. "Gastrointestinal Tract Cancers." In Casciato DA, and Lowitz BB, eds. *Manual of Clinical Oncology*, 4th ed. Philadelphia, PA: Lippincott Williams & Wilkins, 2000: 182–194.

5. Sweed MR, and Meropol NJ. "Assessment, Diagnosis, and Staging." In Berg, D, ed. *Contemporary Issues in Colorectal Cander: A Nursing Perspective.* Boston, MA: Jones and Bartlett Publishers, 2001: 65–79.

6. Fitzpatrick TB, Johnson RA, and Wolf K, eds. "Skin Signs of Systemic Cancers." In *Color Atlas and Synopsis of Clinical Dermatology: Common and Serious Diseases*, 3rd ed. New York, NY: McGraw-Hill, 1997: 504–522.

7. Weiss P, and O'Rourke M. "Cutaneous Paraneoplastic Syndromes." *Clin J Oncol Nurs.* 2000; 4: 257–261.

8. Blanke CD, and Washington K. "Paraneoplastic Phenomena Associated with Gastrointestinal Cancer." In Raghavan D, Brecher ML, and Johnson DH, eds. *Textbook of Uncommon Cancer*, 2nd ed. Chichester, England: John Wiley & Sons, 1999: 469–481.

9. Nicoll D, McPhee S, Chou T, *et al.* "Common Laboratory Tests: Selection and Interpretation." In Nicoll D, McPhee SJ, Chou TM, *et al.*, eds. *Pocket Guide to Diagnostic Tests.* Stamford, CT: Appleton & Lange, 1997: 64.

10. Wu S, Hoshino DF, Zhou A, *et al.* "Practical Approaches to Molecular Screening of Colon Cancer." In Srivastava S, Lippman S, Hong W, *et al.*, eds. *Early Detection of Cancer: Molecular Markers.* Armonk, New York: Futura Publishing, 1994: 237–253.

11. Minamoto T, Mai M, and Ronai Z. "K-*ras* Mutation: Early Detection in Molecular Diagnosis and Risk Assessment of Colorectal, Pancreas, and Lung Cancers— A Review." *Cancer Detect Prev.* 2000; 24: 1–12.

12. Macdonald JS. "Carcinoembryonic Antigen Screening: Pros and Cons." *Semin Oncol.* 1999; 26: 556–560.

13. Desch CE, Benson AB, Smith TJ, *et al.* "Recommended Colorectal Cancer Surveillance Guidelines by the American Society of Clinical Oncology." *J Clin Oncol.* 1999; 17: 1312–1321.

14. Bast RC, Ravdin P, Hayes DF, Bates S, Fritsche H, Jessup JM, Kemeny N, Locker GY, Mennel RG, and Somerfield MR. "2000 Update of Recommendations for the Use of Tumor Markers in Breast and Colorectal Cancer: Clinical Practice Guidelines of the American Society of Clinical Oncology. *Journal of Clinical Oncology.* 2001; 19(6): 1865–1878.

15. Heneghan JP, Salem RR, Lange RC, *et al.* "Transrectal Sonography in Staging Rectal Carcinoma: The Role of Gray-Scale, Colorflow, and Doppler Imaging Analysis." *AJR Am J Roentgenol.* 1997; 169: 124.

16. Schwartz LH. "Advances in Cross-sectional Imaging of Colorectal Cancer." *Semin Oncol.* 1999; 26: 569–576.

17. National Comprehensive Cancer Network. Colon and Rectal Cancer Treatment Guidelines for Patients. NCCN and ACS. 2000, version 1.

18. Akhurst T, Larson SM. "Positron Emission Tomography Imaging of Colorectal Cancer." *Semin Oncol.* 1999; 26: 577–583.

19. Ellenhorn JDI, Coia LR, Alberts SR, and Hoff PM. "Colorectal and Anal Cancers." In Pazdur R, Coia LR, Hoskins HJ, and Wagman LD, eds. *Cancer Management: A Multidisciplinary Approach*, 6th ed. Melville, NY: PRR, Inc, 2002: 295–318.

20. Le Voyer TE, Sigurdson ER, Hanlon AL, *et al.* "Colon Cancer Survival Is Associated with Increasing Number of Lymph Nodes Removed." A Secondary Analysis of INT-0089. *Proceedings of the American Society of Clinical Oncologists*, 2000; 19: 925 (abstr).

21. Greene FL, Page DL, Fleming ID, Fritz AG, Balch CM, Haller DG, and Morrow M. eds. *American Joint Committee on Cancer Staging Manual*, 6th ed. *Colorectal Cancer.* New York, NY: Springer. 2002: 113–123.

PART III

Primary Cancer of the Colon and Rectum: Therapeutic Approaches and Nursing Care

7

Surgical Aspects

Introduction

Surgery is the only potentially curable therapeutic option for patients with cancers of the colon or rectum. Depending on location, lesions may be removed endoscopically, laparoscopically, or by open laparotomy. It is essential that nurses caring for these patients understand their physical and emotional needs, as well as the special needs associated with each surgical procedure.[1]

Surgical Techniques in Colorectal Cancer (CRC)

❖ Polypectomy

❖ Laparoscopic colectomy

❖ Sentinel lymph node biopsy (SLNB)

❖ Open colectomy

❖ Treatment of colon tumors

❖ Treatment of rectal tumors

Management of Polyps—Polypectomy

❖ New polyps can be snared and excised during the sigmoidoscopy and/or colonoscopy.

❖ Individuals with polyps found at sigmoidoscopy should undergo a colonoscopy to check for additional polyps within other colon segments.

  ❖ Benign polyps should be excised with a repeat colonoscopy in 1 year, if negative repeat again at 3 to 5 years.[2]

  ❖ If cancer is present, confined within the head of the polyp, and if there are clear margins, no additional treatment is required.

  ❖ Routine surveillance, however, is necessary: repeat colonoscopy at 1 year. A positive repeat test will require polyp excision, management based on the characteristics of the tumor, and repeat colonoscopy in 1 year. If the test is negative, repeat the colonoscopy in 3 to 5 years.[3]

  ❖ If the tumor has inadequate margins or if it is a sessile polyp with an invasive cancer, surgery to remove all disease is required.[4]

Laparoscopic Colectomy

❖ This alternative to open abdominal colectomy utilizes several small incisions, a videoscope, and TV monitors to assist in the operation.

❖ This method is frequently used to surgically remove cancerous polyps, because it is considered as safe and effective as open colectomy.[5]

❖ The National Cancer Institute (NCI) is sponsoring a large randomized clinical trial to assess the frequency of treatment-related early and late side effects, 30-day mortality, differences in cost effectiveness, disease-free, and overall survival compared with open colectomy.[6]

　❖ A recent interim report of this study noted that patients did experience a slightly shorter hospital stay and less postoperative pain medication, but quality of life and certain complaints (e.g., pain and nausea) during the first two postoperative months were the same.[6]

❖ At this time, the laparoscopic procedure is still considered investigational, because its impact on staging, patterns of recurrence, and survival are not known. The National Comprehensive Cancer Network (NCCN) guidelines do not recommend this procedure unless it is performed in the context of a well-designed clinical trial.[7]

Sentinel Lymph Node Biospy (SLNB)

❖ Identifies the lymph nodes most likely to contain metastatic disease

❖ Procedure: During colectomy, Lymphazurin blue dye is injected around the primary tumor. The dye will drain to the main lymph node(s) (sentinel node) to which cancer cells are most likely to spread first. The sentinel node(s) will appear blue-stained. After lymphadenectomy of the sentinel node(s), pathologic analysis will identify any presence of cancerous cells, increasing the accuracy of staging and thereby providing the best treatment options to improve survival.

❖ Researchers are exploring the use of this technique. Thus far, SLN mapping is proving to be feasible in CRC patients, with an accuracy of more than 95%.[8]

❖ Further prospective clinical trials are needed to evaluate long-term survival.

Open Colectomy

❖ The specific procedure depends on the tumor location within the colon.

❖ The surgical plan is to remove the bowel segment containing the tumor and the corresponding mesentery, and to maximize the removal of regional lymph nodes, while maintaining function.[9] The amount of colon removed depends on the mesenteric nodal resection.[10]

❖ Five basic principles governing CRC resections.[5]
  ❖ Opportunity for a full intra-abdominal assessment
  ❖ Identification of visceral metastases
  ❖ Safe creation of an stoma, where applicable
  ❖ Adequate longitudinal and radial margins of resection
    1. 5-cm of normal bowel on either side of the tumor is ideal, but 2-cm margins may be sat-

isfactory if there is an adequate mesentery resection[3]

❖ Ensurance of full mesenteric and nodal dissections

Treatment of Cancers in the Right Colon: Ascending, Transverse, and Descending Colon

❖ A right or extended right colectomy

  ❖ Candidates: individuals with uncomplicated carcinomas of the right colon, hepatic flexure, and transverse colon

  ❖ Procedure: Illustrated in Figure 7-1. The ileum and left transverse colon are anastomosed.[3] Care is made not to remove more than 50 cm to minimize the effects on vitamin B12 (may cause anemia) and bile salt absorption (may result in malabsorption of nutrients and/or chronic diarrhea).[11]

❖ A transverse colectomy or an extended right hemicolectomy

  ❖ Candidates: individuals with tumors in the mid-transverse colon

  ❖ Procedure–transverse colectomy: Illustrated in Figure 7-2. Anastomosis of the ascending and descending colons[12] follows removal of the colon segments.

FIGURE 7-1
Right colectomy

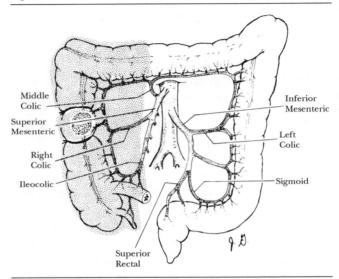

Middle Colic

Superior Mesenteric

Right Colic

Ileocolic

Inferior Mesenteric

Left Colic

Sigmoid

Superior Rectal

Source: Hoebler L. "Colon and Rectal Cancer." In Groenwald SL, Frogge MH, Goodman M, *et al. Cancer Nursing: Principles and Practice*, 4th ed. Boston, MA: Jones & Bartlett, 1997: 1036–1054.

❖ Procedure—extended right hemicolectomy: Illustrated in Figure 7-3. The ileum and proximal descending colon are anastomosed. This is the preferred procedure for elderly patients, where there is concern about a well-vascularized anastomosis.[12]

FIGURE 7-2
Transverse colectomy

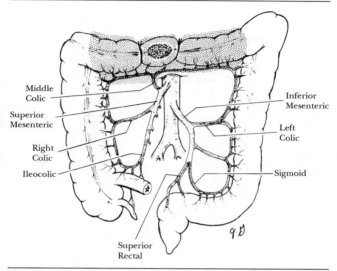

Middle
Colic

Superior
Mesenteric

Right
Colic

Ileocolic

Superior
Rectal

Inferior
Mesenteric

Left
Colic

Sigmoid

Source: Hoebler L. "Colon and Rectal Cancer." In Groenwald SL, Frogge MH, Goodman M, *et al. Cancer Nursing: Principles and Practice*, 4th ed. Boston, MA: Jones & Bartlett, 1997: 1036–1054.

Treatment of Cancers in the Left Colon

❖ A left colectomy

 ❖ Candidates: individuals with uncomplicated tumors in the splenic flexure and the descending colon

FIGURE 7–3
Extended resection for transverse colon carcinoma

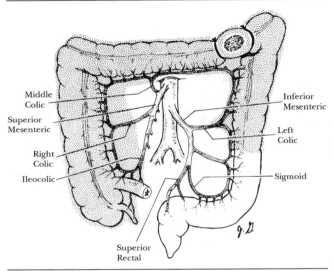

Source: Hoebler L. "Colon and Rectal Cancer." In Groenwald SL, Frogge MH, Goodman M, *et al. Cancer Nursing: Principles and Practice*, 4th ed. Boston, MA: Jones & Bartlett, 1997: 1036–1054.

- ❖ Procedure for a splenic flexure lesion:
  Illustrated in Figure 7-4. The right transverse
  colon and the sigmoid colon are anastomosed.
- ❖ Procedure for a descending colon lesion:
  Illustrated in Figure 7.5. The right transverse
  colon and distal sigmoid colon are anastomosed.

FIGURE 7-4
Colectomy for splenic flexure carcinoma

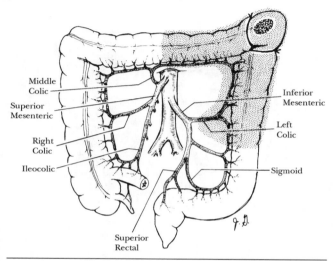

Source: Hoebler L. "Colon and Rectal Cancer." In Groenwald SL, Frogge MH, Goodman M, *et al. Cancer Nursing: Principles and Practice*, 4th ed. Boston, MA: Jones & Bartlett, 1997: 1036-1054.

- ❖ Sigmoid colectomy
    - ❖ Candidates: individuals with uncomplicated lesions in the sigmoid, rectosigmoid, and upper rectum
    - ❖ Procedure: An anterior resection with preservation of the sympathetic nerves (Illustrated in Figure 7.6). The descending colon and upper rectum are anastomosed.

FIGURE 7-5
Left colectomy

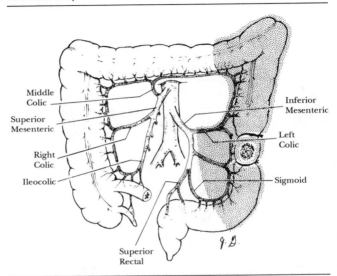

Middle Colic

Superior Mesenteric

Right Colic

Ileocolic

Inferior Mesenteric

Left Colic

Sigmoid

Superior Rectal

Source: Hoebler L. "Colon and Rectal Cancer." In Groenwald SL, Frogge MH, Goodman M, *et al. Cancer Nursing: Principles and Practice*, 4th ed. Boston, MA: Jones & Bartlett, 1997: 1036–1054.

Treatment of Obstructing Tumors

❖ May require one of three approaches

  ❖ Either a two-stage or a traditional three-stage surgical approach

  1. The two-stage (Hartmann) procedure: the tumor is resected, the proximal colon is brought to the skin as an end-colostomy,

FIGURE 7-6
Sigmoid colectomy

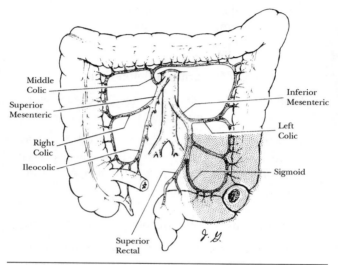

Source: Hoebler L. "Colon and Rectal Cancer." In Groenwald SL, Frogge MH, Goodman M, *et al. Cancer Nursing: Principles and Practice*, 4th ed. Boston, MA: Jones & Bartlett, 1997: 1036–1054.

and the distal colon is sutured or stapled closed; a second operation follows several months later to reverse the colostomy and reestablish intestinal continuity.

2. The traditional three-stage procedure (primarily for tumors in the left-colon) involves the creation of diverting transverse colostomy or a cecostomy (for decompression), followed by a tumor resection 10 to 14 days later, and then several months later a reversal of the

colostomy and reestablishment of intestinal continuity.[13]

* A resection with a permanent stoma
* A resection, intraoperative bowel lavage, and primary anastomosis

Treatment of Perforating Colon Cancer

❖ Sealed, perforated tumors may be resected with an end-to-end anastomosis.

❖ Open perforations are generally resected with a proximal colostomy, followed later by a reversal of the colostomy and reestablishment of intestinal continuity.[10]

Treatment of Lesions Invading Adjacent Organs

❖ Procedure: resection of the adherent or invaded organ along with resection of the primary tumor, followed by an end-to-end anastomosis

Treatment of Rectal Cancers

❖ Surgical options depend on depth of invasion into the rectal wall, the size and gross appearance of the cancer, presence or absence of regional lymph node involvement, and distance above the anal verge.[12] Bowel function status and issues regarding re-anostomosis are also considered

❖ Surgical procedures
   * Local excision

❖ Anterior resection
❖ Sphincter-preserving abdominal surgery
❖ Abdominoperineal resection

Local Excision (Transanal Excision)

❖ Candidates: individuals with rectal tumors above 5 cm from the anal verge which are well-differentiated, limited to the submucosa, less than 3 to 4 cm in diameter, and complete excision with negative margins is possible.

❖ Procedure: The tissue including the tumor is resected including a 1-cm clear margin and perirectal fat (excised to assess for lymph node involvement).[13]

Anterior Resection with Mesorectal Excision

❖ Candidates: individuals with tumors in the middle and upper rectum (6 to 15 cm from the anal verge; must have a least 5 cm of rectum below the tumor)[6]

❖ Procedure: A segment of bowel above and below the tumor is removed; the remaining section of the left colon is pulled down to meet the remaining rectum forming an end-to-end anastomosis[14] (Figure 7.7).

FIGURE 7-7
Anterior rectal resection

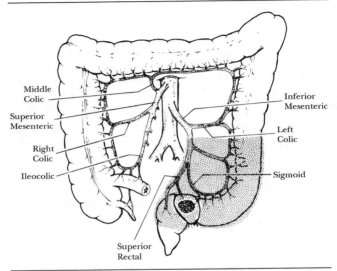

Middle Colic

Superior Mesenteric

Right Colic

Ileocolic

Inferior Mesenteric

Left Colic

Sigmoid

Superior Rectal

Source: Hoebler L. "Colon and Rectal Cancer." In Groenwald SL, Frogge MH, Goodman M, *et al. Cancer Nursing: Principles and Practice*, 4th ed. Boston, MA: Jones & Bartlett, 1997: 1036–1054.

Sphincter Preserving Abdominal Surgery: Low Anterior Resection ([LAR] with Total Mesorectal Excision/Coloanal Anastomosis

❖ Considered by many to be the standard surgery for patients with cancer in the middle rectum and some distal rectal lesions, except those too close to the anal verge.

❖ Candidates: individuals with uncomplicated tumors of the middle and lower rectum (about 6 cm to 15 cm above the anal verge)[9]

❖ Procedure: removal of bowel above and below the lesion with coloanal anastomosis and with preservation of the sympathetic and parasympathetic nerves (Figure 7–7)[14]

　❖ Dissection performed below the peritoneal reflection with at least a 2 cm distal margin for anostomosis.

　❖ The anastomosis sometimes involves a colopouch, a coloanal sleeve anastomosis, or if possible, an end-to-end anastomosis.[14]

　❖ The anastomosis must have an excellent blood supply with no tension, and there must be adequate sphincter muscle function.[1]

Abdominoperineal Resection (APR)

❖ Standard procedure for patients with lesions in the lower rectum

❖ Candidates: individuals with involvement of the sphincter muscles, rectovaginal septum, or if the tumor extends to within 2 cm of the dentate line

❖ Procedure: a two-phased operation performed both within the abdomen and from the rectal area. From the abdomen, the colon and rectum are freed from the mesentery; then from the rectal area, the entire rectum, including the tumor and surrounding lymph nodes and tissue, is removed. This often results in a large wound, which takes several weeks or months to heal. The patient will also have a permanent colostomy[14] (Figure 7–8).

FIGURE 7–8
Abdominoperineal resection

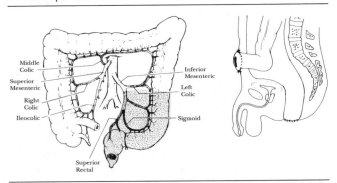

Source: Hoebler L. "Colon and Rectal Cancer." In Groenwald SL, Frogge MH, Goodman M, *et al. Cancer Nursing: Principles and Practice*, 4th ed. Boston, MA: Jones & Bartlett, 1997: 1036–1054.

Ostomy Management

❖ The terms *ostomy* and *stoma* are often used interchangeably though they are different.

  ❖ An ostomy is a surgical opening in the body for diversion of body waste.

  ❖ A stoma is the actual end of the ureter, small or large bowel seen protruding through the abdominal wall.[15]

  ❖ Most common type of ostomy for patients with CRC is the colostomy. It may be temporary or permanent. It maybe "named" for the section of colon from which it is created, e.g., sigmoid colostomy. Other types of ostomies include an ileostomy and ileoanal anastomosis (J-pouch).

❖ Types of ostomy interventions

  ❖ There are two types of intestinal ostomies: a colostomy and ileostomy.

    1. The placement of the intestinal ostomy depends on the specific area proximal to the cancerous lesion. The consistency of the output of a colostomy depends on the location of the ostomy.[1]

  ❖ Ileostomy is a surgical opening made in the abdominal wall for the elimination of digested food from the small intestine, usually from the distal small bowel or terminal ileum. These are usually placed in the right lower abdominal quadrant.[16] Drainage from an ileostomy is watery.

  ❖ Colostomy is a surgical opening made in the abdominal wall for the elimination of digested food from the large intestine; it is commonly performed along the colon from the cecum to the sigmoid colon.[15]

    1. A cecostomy and ascending colostomy is placed in the right lower abdominal quadrant and produces a mixture of mushy stool and water.

    2. Transverse colostomies are placed on either the left or right upper abdominal quadrant and produce mushy to semiformed stool.[1]

    3. Descending colon and sigmoid colostomies are located in the left lower quadrant and produce semiformed to formed stool.[16]

4. Ileoanal anastomosis (J-pouch). This is not really an ostomy, but rather an anastomotic procedure that creates an internal pouch from a section of the terminal ileum. A hole is cut in the bottom of the "pouch," and this is connected to the anus. The sphincter muscles control continence. This procedure may be performed in patients with a history of ulcerative colitis or familial adenomatous polyposis.[15]

❖ Three common surgical constructions of a stoma: end, loop, and double barrel[16]

1. An end stoma is formed when the proximal resected end of the colon is brought out to the abdominal surface. The distal portion of the colon is often removed. This is usually a permanent procedure.[16]

2. A loop stoma is formed when a loop of colon is brought out to the abdominal surface. An opening is cut in the loop. This stoma is produced to rest the bowel and is often temporary; it is reversible at a later point.[16]

3. A double-barrel stoma is formed when both ends of the freshly cut colon are brought out to the abdominal surface; note, this means there are two stomas.[16] The proximal stoma drains bowel contents; the distal end will occasionally discharge mucous produced from the lower portion of the bowel.

❖ Preoperative preparation for an ostomy procedure

   ❖ Meet with an enterstomal therapy nurse (CWOCN)

   1. Goals: preoperative teaching and siting of the stoma[16,17]

   2. Siting of the stoma is done after completing a past medical history and a comprehensive assessment of the abdominal area to determine the best site for the ostomy avoiding folds or creases of the abdomen. Once the site is selected, it is marked with a nontoxic marker and covered with a transparent dressing to prevent the area from being scrubbed and the markings erased.

   ❖ In the case of emergency surgery, preoperative placement of the stoma may not be possible.[16]

   ❖ Factors to consider regarding an individual's ability to independently care for an ostomy: mental status, hand dexterity, vision, coordination, and emotional acceptance of the procedure. Age alone is not a deciding factor.

   ❖ Some common preoperative concerns include fear of an ostomy malfunction (e.g., stool leakage), odor, self-image, care of the ostomy, ability to participate in social activities, sports, and sexual intercourse.[18]

   ❖ Education can be key to acceptance of the ostomy, which can also be influenced by ease of care.

❖ Postoperative considerations and care

❖ Enterostomal therapy nurse reinforces information, provides emotional support, and assists in selection of appliances.

❖ Early participation in care is important for the patient's adjustment.[1,17,18]

❖ Initially, a one-piece appliance system is placed around the stoma. This type of system is used until the area heals and becomes less tender. Eventually, a two-piece system may be used if easier for the patient.

❖ The patient can expect the stoma to drain mucous and blood exudate into the pouching system for 3 to 5 days. As the diet increases from liquid to solid foods, the output becomes thicker with the final thickness depending on the placement along the colon. The proximal portion of the bowel returns to "normal" function within 3 to 5 days. Flatulence also begins to escape through the stoma; therefore, the bag will need to be opened occasionally during the day to release the air.

❖ Selection of products (appliances)

1. Choice of appliances depends on the location of the stoma site, drainage consistency, peristomal skin condition, and the condition of the stoma.

2. Correct fit of the appliance is crucial in preventing leakage of the fecal fluid.

3. Pouching systems vary.

a. All have faceplates (flanges) that make contact with the skin surface. The flange may be a skin barrier wafer, an adhesive surface, or a synthetic surface. It may be flat or convex; stationary or floating; a pre-cut or cut-to-fit system; or a one-piece (bag and flange are attached) or two-piece (bag and flange are separate pieces) system.[1]

b. Bag options are more limited, but include the length, type of backing, and whether it contains a filter to automatically release flatulence.

c. Skin barriers, used to protect the skin from the appliance and fecal leakage, are also varied. Some products have an alcohol base and can cause stinging if there are any open areas on the skin.[1]

d. Allergies to plastic, latex, pectin or tape backings may cause skin erosion, blistering, or seepage or peeling at the contact surface, usually the epidermal level of the skin, or cause the appliance to become prematurely disconnected.[1]

❖ Directions for changing the ostomy bag and flange are outlined in Chapter 13.

Nursing Care of Patients with Bowel Surgery

❖ Preoperative preparation (*note:* done entirely at home)

  ❖ Starting the day before the operation the patient will start a regime of mechanical cleansing and antibiotic administration to prevent wound infection and intra-abdominal abscess formation.

  ❖ Options for mechanical cleansing:[1]

   1. Drink a bottle of Fleet's phospha sode and 24 oz of clear liquid at 12 P.M. and 6 P.M. on the day before surgery.
   2. Drink approximately 4 L Go-Lytely or Co-Lyte over a period of 4 hours. Refrigerating the liquid can make it more palatable.

  ❖ Common antibiotic regimen: 1 g each of neomycin sulfate and erythromycin at 1 P.M., 2 P.M., and 11 P.M. on the day before surgery and an intravenous broad-spectrum antibiotic immediately before surgery.

  ❖ The patient is then NPO (nothing by mouth) after midnight.

  ❖ The next morning the patient is admitted to the hospital for surgery. In-depth preoperative education is frequently done in the surgeon's office. After admission to the hospital, it is important to reinforce information and treatment recommendations and answer any questions.

❖ Postoperative care

  ❖ Attention is focused on preventing complications and promoting convalescence.

  1. Potential complications of a colectomy: atelectasis or pneumonia, pain, fluid and electrolyte imbalances, leakage from the anastomotic site, poor wound healing, abdominal distention, paralytic ileus, inadequate dietary intake, and weight loss. Potential additional complications of an abdominoperinal resection: urinary retention and impotence

  ❖ Hospital duration is about 4 to 6 days with an open colectomy, slightly shorter with a laparoscopic colectomy.

  ❖ Education focuses on self-care after discharge: wound care, prevention of infection, pain management, prevention of thromboses, importance of adequate nutrition and fluid intake, review plans for surgical and medical follow-up, and if applicable, ostomy care.

References

1. Waldman AR, and Crane ME. "Surgical Aspects of Colon Cancer." In Berg, DT, ed. *Contemporary Issues in Colorectal Cancer: A Nursing Perspective.* Boston, MA: Jones and Bartlett Publishers, 2001: 105–134.

2. American Cancer Society. "American Cancer Society Guidelines on Screening and Surveillance for the Early Detection of Adenomatous Polyps and Colorectal

Cancer—Update 2001." *CA: A Cancer Journal for Clinicians*. January/February 2001. 51 (1): 44–54.

3. Kodner IJ, Fry RD, Fleshman JW, *et al.* "Colon, Rectum, and Anus." In Schwartz SI, *et al.*, eds. *Principles of Surgery*, 7th ed. New York, NY: McGraw-Hill, 1999: 1265–1382.

4. Eckhauser FE, and Knol JA. "Surgery for Primary and Metastatic Colorectal Cancer." *Gastroenterol Clin North Am.* 1997; 26: 103–128.

5. Greene F. "Laparoscopic Management of Colorectal Cancer." *CA Cancer J Clin.* 1999; 49: 221–228.

6. National Cancer Institute. Colon and Rectal Cancer Homepage. Available at http://www.cancer.gov/cancer-information/cancer-type/colon-and-rectal/. Accessed June 30, 2002.

7. National Comprehensive Cancer Network (NCCN). "Colon and Rectal Cancer Treatment Guidelines." In *The Complete Library of Practice Guidelines in Oncology*, 2nd ed. Version 2001. Rockledge, PA: NCCN, 2001.

8. Saha S, Wiese D, Badin J, *et al.* "Technical Details of Sentinel Lymph Node Mapping in Colorectal Cancer and Its Impact on Staging." *Ann Surg Oncol.* 2000; 7: 120–124.

9. Ellenhorn JDI, Coia LR, Alberts SR, and Hoff PM. "Colorectal and Anal Cancers." In Pazdur R, Coia LR, Hoskins HJ, and Wagman LD, eds. *Cancer Management: A Multidisciplinary Approach*, 6th ed. Melville, NY: PRR, Inc, 2002: 295–318.

10. Goldberg RM. "Gastrointestinal Tract Cancers." In Casciato DA and Lowitz BB, eds. *Manual of Clinical Oncology*, 4th ed. Philadelphia, PA: Lippincott Williams & Wilkins, 2000: 182–194.

11. Kettlewell MG. "Colorectal Cancer and Benign

Tumours of the Colon." In Morris PJ, and Malt RA, eds. *Oxford Textbook of Surgery*. New York: Oxford University Press, 1994: 1060–1087.

12. Bleday R, and Steele G. "Colorectal Cancer Surgery." In Rustgi AK, ed. *Gastrointestinal Cancers: Biology, Diagnosis, and Therapy*. Philadelphia, PA: Lippincott-Raven Publishers, 1995: 455–475.

13. Guillem JG, and Cohen AM. "Current issues in colorectal cancer surgery." *Semin Oncol*. 1999; 26: 505–513.

14. Texas Cancer Center. Your Guide to Limited Surgery in the Treatment of Cancer. Available at http://www.hern.org/~dick/rectal/treatment.html. Accessed June 30, 2002.

15. United Ostomy Association. "Key Ostomy Terms and UOA Fact Sheets." February 26, 2002. Available at http://www.uoa.org/ostomyinfo.shtml. Accessed June 30, 2002.

16. Hampton BG, and Bryant R. *Ostomies and Continent Diversions*. St. Louis, MO: Mosby–Year Book, 1992: 1–128.

17. Piwonka MA, and Merino J. "A Multidimensional Modeling of Predictors Influencing the Adjustment to a Colostomy." *JWOCN*. 1999; 26: 298–305.

18. Pieper B, and Mikols C. "Predischarge and Postdischarge Concerns of Persons with an Ostomy." *JWOCN*. 1996; 23: 105–109.

8

Radiation Therapy

Introduction

Radiation therapy is an important modality in the treatment of colorectal cancers, especially those in the rectal area. This modality may be used alone or in combination with surgery and/or chemotherapy. Nursing management is essential to the quality of life for patients undergoing radiation therapy.

- ❖ Radiation therapy is the use of ionizing radiation to destroy cancer cells.[1]

  - ❖ The radiation therapy treatment team is a multidisciplinary group including radiation oncologist, radiation therapist, medical physicist, dosimetrist, and nurse. Often social workers, dietitians, clinical trials staff, and cancer patient support programs are available.
  - ❖ The goal of radiation therapy is to deliver a therapeutic dose of ionizing radiation to the tumor while minimizing injury to surrounding healthy tissues.[1]

Principles of External Beam Radiation Therapy in the Treatment of CRC

❖ Depending on stage of disease and prognostic factors, radiation may be given in a neoadjuvant or adjuvant setting. In either setting it may also be given in combination with chemotherapy.

  ❖ Neoadjuvant—goal: reduce tumor burden (downstage the tumor) to improve resectability and decrease chance of needing a permanent colostomy

  ❖ Adjuvant—goal: eradicate remaining cancer cells and reduce the risk of local recurrence

❖ The linear accelerator (linac) is the most common treatment-delivery machine for external beam radiation therapy. Patients with CRC are primarily treated with particulate radiation (high-energy photons), which have a limited ability to penetrate into deep tissues.

❖ Dose delivery

  ❖ Fractionation: one fraction of the total treatment dose is administered once a day over a prescribed number of days or weeks

  ❖ Hyperfractionation: more than one fraction a day of the total treatment dose

  ❖ Multi-field treatment plan: the treatment beam is directed at the tumor from three or four different directions, a combination of front, back, left or right side. For example if the beam is directed from three directions, it would be called a three-field treatment plan. This treatment provides appropriate therapy to the tumor site, but by rotating the radiation, the surrounding normal tissues are spared the full dose and the potential toxicities.

❖ All appropriate measures are used to ensure that the patient's treatment is reproduced exactly at each session.

❖ In CRC, one fixed dose (fraction) of radiation therapy is usually administered each day in a three-field or four-field treatment plan.

Steps in the Radiation Treatment Process

❖ Before radiation therapy can be safely administered, several essential steps must take place.

❖ Pretreatment evaluation and studies

  ❖ The patient, and ideally the significant others, meet with the radiation oncologist to discuss the role of radiation therapy and the specific treatment plan. During this consultation, a thorough history and physical examination are completed while diagnostic and laboratory tests are completed and/or reviewed to confirm the diagnosis and tumor location and size.

  1. Common diagnostic and laboratory tests include computed tomography (CT) scan or magnetic resonance imaging (MRI) of the abdomen and pelvis, chest x-ray, transrectal ultrasound, carcinoembryonic antigen (CEA), complete blood count, serum chemistry, liver function tests, and pathology reports.

* ❖ The patient and significant other(s) also meet with the radiation therapy nurse who provides them with additional details pertinent to the treatment plan—side effects, and symptom management measures. Information is provided in a manner consistent with their educational and cultural backgrounds.

❖ Treatment planning

* ❖ The treatment planning is initiated once the decision has been made to include radiation therapy in the overall treatment plan.
* ❖ Goal of treatment planning is to define the target volume to be treated yet minimize the dose of radiation to healthy tissue/organs in the surrounding area.
* ❖ The patient's age, performance status, prognosis, stage of disease, tumor histology, tumor size, tumor location, known patterns of metastatic spread, possible side effects, and available treatment equipment are also taken into consideration during the treatment planning stage.

❖ Simulation

* ❖ This appointment is an enactment of the actual radiation therapy treatment visit, but no radiation is delivered. The appointment lasts about one hour. It is during simulation that the specific treatment area(s) to be shielded are precisely defined.

- ❖ Barium as well as several other procedures may be used to provide better visualization of the small bowel, vagina, bladder, rectum, and anus. These procedures provide information that will help minimize toxicity and better delineate the treatment area. Immobilization devices, including lead blocks, are typically used in patients with CRC to shield specific body areas.
- ❖ During simulation, and during the actual treatments, the patient lies prone on the treatment table (also called treatment couch). The patient is draped to expose the treatment area. Radiographic x-rays (portal films) are taken and used to isolate the tumor, identify normal tissues that will be part of the treatment field, and determine the treatment volume. These films are also used during treatments to ensure reproducibility of the treatment field. Once the treatment field has been defined, skin markings or tattoos are applied to the skin to serve as landmarks.
- ❖ All of the information from the treatment planning and simulation visits allows the physicist and dosimetrist to precisely formulate the actual treatment dose.

- ❖ Treatment days
  - ❖ The external radiation therapy dose is typically delivered once a day, Monday through Friday. The treatment takes only 3 to 5 minutes, but the patient is in the treatment room for 10 to 15 minutes so they can be properly positioned.

* At least once weekly the patient meets with the radiation oncologist and nurse to assess how they are responding to the treatment. Reinforcement of self-care measures, symptomatic strategies, and other educational needs are addressed at this time.

Treatment of Colon Cancer

* National Comprehensive Cancer Network (NCCN) guidelines for the adjuvant treatment of patients with colon cancer:[2]
    * T1-3 N1-2 M0 disease: systemic chemotherapy with 5-fluorouracil (5-FU) and leucovorin, or 5-FU, leucovorin, and radiation, if perforation is present[2]
    * T4 N1-2 M0 disease: 5-FU and leucovorin with or without radiation[2]
    * Adjuvant radiation therapy for colon cancer should be given only in the context of a well designed, prospective clinical trial.[3]
* Sample radiation regimen for locally advanced colon cancer
    * The typical daily postoperative dose is 180 cGy for 25 fractions with a boost dose of 180 cGy for 3 fractions to the postoperative site. This results in a total dose of 5,040 cGy.
* Radiation therapy for metastatic colon cancer— The treatment goal is palliative, and therefore, the dose and treatment fields vary, based on the site of disease.

Treatment of Rectal Cancer

General Considerations

❖ Combined modality therapy (chemotherapy plus radiotherapy) requires coordination of care between medical and radiation therapy, regardless of the sequence of each modality.

❖ Considerations: scheduling and logistical issues, communication of treatment plans, patient education, and clarifying roles to the patient and family

❖ The chemotherapy is often 5-fluorouracil (5-FU) based and is given either intermittently or by continuous infusion.

❖ Postoperative radiotherapy is more commonly administered as compared with preoperative therapy, approximately 75% and 22% respectively.[4]

Preoperative Radiotherapy

❖ Potential advantages
  ❖ Reduced volume of tumor, decreased tumor seeding, less acute toxicity, increased radiosensitivity, and enhanced sphincter preservation[5]

❖ Potential disadvantage
  ❖ Theoretical overtreatment of about 10% to 15% of patients with T1-2 N0 M0 disease that would not require adjuvant therapy[6]

❖ Goal: preserve sphincter function

❖ Two recent studies have confirmed the benefit of preoperative radiotherapy with a decrease in local recurrence and an improvement in overall survival.[5] Research also demonstrates that the toxicity of preoperative combined modality regimens is less than when the chemotherapy is given with postoperative radiation therapy.[7]

❖ Preoperative treatment of rectal cancer

• The typical dose is 180 cGy over 25 fractions to a total dose of 4,500 cGy. A "boost or cone down" dose is also often given specifically to the primary area of disease plus a 2- to 3-cm margin about it. The dose is 180 cGy over 3 fractions to a total of 540 cGy. The results in a total preoperative treatment dose of 5,040 cGy over 5 to 6 weeks. Surgery is usually scheduled 4 to 6 weeks after the radiation therapy is completed.

Postoperative Radiotherapy

❖ Potential advantages
   ❖ Only those patients who need radiotherapy receive it.
   ❖ The application of surgical clips during surgery can accurately define the tumor bed.[8]

❖ Goals: improve local tumor control, decrease distant metastais, and improve survival[5]

❖ Though postoperative radiotherapy is used more often, clinical trials have shown little advantage in local control and a markedly inferior rate of sphincter control as compared with surgery alone.[8,9]

❖ Postoperative treatment of rectal cancer

* The typical dose may be higher depending on
  the institution. Radiation therapy is started 4 to
  6 weeks after surgery.

NCCN Guidelines for the Treatment of Rectal Cancer

❖ T1-2 N0 M0 surgery followed by observation

❖ T1-2 N1-2 M0, or T3 N0-2 M0: preoperative 5-FU
  plus radiotherapy before surgery, followed by systemic 5-FU with or without leucovorin postoperatively for four cycles. If the patient does not
  receive neoadjuvant therapy, NCCN recommends
  5-FU with or without leucovorin given postoperatively for two cycles, followed by 5-FU and radiotherapy, and then two additional cycles of 5-FU
  with or without leucovorin.[2]

❖ For any T4 disease: continuous or intermittent
  systemic infusion of 5-FU with or without leucovorin and preoperative radiotherapy, followed by
  surgery if resection is possible, then four additional cycles of 5-FU with or without leucovorin[2]

Combined Modality Therapy

❖ A decline in local recurrence, a decrease in
  metastatic spread, and a significant improvement
  in survival have been demonstrated with the combination of standard radiation and 5-FU-based
  chemotherapy as compared with radiation therapy
  alone in patients with resectable rectal cancer.[5,10]

- Most combined-modality therapy regimens include six cycles of 5-FU-based chemotherapy plus concurrent pelvic radiation.[5,11]

❖ The majority of patients with rectosigmoid and rectal cancer are treated with combined-modality regimens.[4]

Side Effects of External Beam Radiotherapy

❖ Side effects may be classified as either acute or chronic.
  - ❖ Acute side effects arise during treatment and up to 6 months after treatment. They often resolve within a few weeks to months after treatment is completed.
  - ❖ Late side effects, often a continuation of the acute effects, arise months to years after treatment is completed.

❖ The side effects associated with radiotherapy are often predictable and based on several common factors:
  - ❖ The treatment site and volume irradiated
  - ❖ The daily dose of radiation
  - ❖ Concomitant therapies
  - ❖ Individual differences

❖ Common acute side effects:[11]
  - ❖ Skin reactions: erythema, dry or moist desquamation, and hyperpigmentation
  - ❖ Diarrhea with or without abdominal cramps, with or without pain

- ❖ Myelosuppression
- ❖ Proctitis
- ❖ Cystitis
- ❖ Fatigue

❖ Common late effects[11]

- ❖ Skin reactions: telangiectasias, fibrosis, and hyper-or hypopigmentation
- ❖ Bowel changes: small bowel obstruction, fibrosis, adhesions, and fistulas
- ❖ Late cystitis, atrophy, organ or sexual dysfunction, ulceration, and necrosis

❖ Patient education considerations:[11]

- ❖ Patient education, reinforcement of symptom management strategies, and emotional support by members of the radiation therapy team, especially the radiation therapy nurse, are not a one-time discussions, but rather an ongoing process.
- ❖ It is important to reinforce two key messages with patients.

  1. Radiation is local therapy not a systemic one, thus the side effects are caused by damage to normal tissue within the treatment field, not elsewhere in the body.
  2. Patients are not radioactive because of radiation therapy treatments.

❖ Specific educational tips:[11]

- ❖ Table 8-1 outlines potential radiation therapy–induced side effects and possible nursing interventions.[11]

TABLE 8–1
Potential Radiation Therapy-Induced Side Effects and Possible Interventions

Side Effect	Onset	Usual Duration	Presentation	Intervention
Erythema	Approximately 2 to 3 weeks after start of treatment.	Resolves within 10 to 14 days after treatment completed.	Skin that is pink or tender. Common in perineal area and gluteal folds.	Position patient in prone position to minimize skin reactions. Use mild cleansing agent to clean area daily and after toileting. Apply unscented moisturizing protective cream, e.g., Aquaphor. Avoid lotions or creams with perfume, talc, metals.
Dry desquamation	Approximately 2 to 3 weeks after the start of treatment.	Resolves approximately 14 days after treatment completed.	Skin is scaling, flaking, pruritic, and sometimes painful.	Use tepid water or a wound cleanser to clean area twice a day and as needed after toileting. Apply unscented protective cream, e.g., Aquaphor. If pruritic, apply topical antihistamine, take cool bath/shower, use systemic pain medications and antihistamines as needed. Assess for fungal infection and treat either topically or systemically. Warn patient not to use cornstarch or steroid creams.

TABLE 8-1
Potential Radiation Therapy-Induced Side Effects and Possible Interventions (continued)

Side Effect	Onset	Usual Duration	Presentation	Intervention
Moist desquamation	Several weeks after the start of therapy.	Resolves 2 to 3 weeks after treatment completed.	Skin is painful, weeping, sloughing, or with abscesses.	Sitz baths, showers, whirlpool treatment as needed to debride skin. Gently cleanse area with drying antibacterial cleanser twice a day and as needed after toileting; pat dry after each cleansing. Apply an unscented protective cream, e.g. Aquaphor. Apply adhesive peripad (pantyliner) to underwear or use diapers. Allow area to be open to air as possible. Moist soaks, e.g., Domeboro Astringent Solution TID x 20 minutes may be considered. Provide pain medications as needed.
Hyperpigmenta-tion	Approximately 2 to 3 weeks after start of treatment.	Resolves slowly.	Mild to deep tanning discoloration.	As for erythema.

(continued)

TABLE 8-1

Potential Radiation Therapy-Induced Side Effects and Possible Interventions (continued)

Side Effect	Onset	Usual Duration	Presentation	Intervention
Itching/folliculitis	Approximately 1 to 2 weeks after start of treatment.	Variable. May not resolve until treatment completed.	Itchy red skin. Small red dots perineal area.	Oatmeal colloidal baths and soaps. Apply unscented moisturizing, protective cream. Antihistamine topically or systemically as needed; especially useful at bedtime.
Fatigue	Initially noticed during the 2nd or 3rd week of treatment.	Peaks near end of therapy and gradually resolves over one week to months after treatment completed.	Increased, often unexplained, tiredness, very common complaint. May be acute or chronic.	Encourage rest periods. Maintain usual exercise level. If did not exercise regularly, walking, with prior approval from the physician, may be helpful. Eat a well-balanced diet. Accept assistance with activities of daily living. Prioritize activities. May need to either work part time or take time off especially towards end of therapy. Transportation assistance can be helpful.

(continued)

TABLE 8-1
Potential Radiation Therapy-Induced Side Effects and Possible Interventions (continued)

Side Effect	Onset	Usual Duration	Presentation	Intervention
Anorexia/nausea	Nausea: 1 to 2 hours after treatment.	Resolve after treatment completed.	Lack of interest in food or desire to eat. Nausea.	Encourage patients not to eat heavy meals prior to treatments. Prescribe an antiemetic prior to therapy and/or on a regular schedule. Commonly prescribed antiemetics include prochlorperazine maleate or the 5HT3 antagonists. Monitor weight several times during week. Refer to a dietitian for weight maintenance suggestions.

(continued)

TABLE 8-1

Potential Radiation Therapy-Induced Side Effects and Possible Interventions (continued)

Side Effect	Onset	Usual Duration	Presentation	Intervention
Diarrhea	May start within 10 to 14 days after start of therapy, earlier if also receiving chemotherapy.	Starts to resolve after therapy completed, but may be prolonged.	Common in the majority of patients. May be an acute or late effect. Increased frequency of liquid or formed stool, abdominal cramping, and tenesmus. Bloating and flatus also reported.	Frequently prescribed antidiarrheal medications: loperamide hydrochloride and diphenoxylate hydrochloride with atropine, or paregoric. Metamucil may be helpful in some patients. Encourage patients to drink 6–8 glasses of nonalcoholic, non-caffeinated fluids each day. Dietary changes (low fiber, fat, lactose) with supplements as tolerated. Fluid and electrolyte replacement as needed. Monitor weight several times during week. Careful cleansing of the perianal area after each stooling. Sitz baths and unscented baby wipes may be helpful. Hydrocortisone may relieve proctitis.

(continued)

TABLE 8-1

Potential Radiation Therapy-Induced Side Effects and Possible Interventions (continued)

Side Effect	Onset	Usual Duration	Presentation	Intervention
Cystitis	Approximately 2 to 3 weeks after the start of therapy.	Slowly resolves after the completion of therapy.	Frequency, dysuria, urgency. Urinary tract infection may occur. In men, inflammation of the prostate with obstructed urine flow is rare.	Encourage drinking 2-3 liters of fluid each day. Dietary changes: avoid caffeine, alcohol, spices, and tobacco. Phenazopyridine hydrochloride may be prescribed as needed for dysuria. Oxybutynin chloride may be helpful for bladder spasms. Antibiotics may be necessary. A foley catheter may be placed in men if there is a reduction in urinary outflow.
Myelosuppression	Approximately 10 to 14 days after start of therapy.	Within 1 to 2 weeks after the nadir.	Leukopenia, thrombocytopenia, anemia.	Monitoring blood counts. Treatment break if leukopenia less than 2/mm3 or platelets less than 75, 000/uL. Monitor temperature during anticipated nadir. Institute bleeding and infection precautions as needed based on blood counts.

Source: Gosselin T. "Radiation Therapy." In Berg, D, ed. *Contemporary Issues in Colorectal Cancer: A Nursing Perspective.* Boston, MA: Jones and Bartlett Publishers, 2001: 135–156.

❖ Skin reactions

1. Postoperative patients are at risk for infection during radiation therapy if the surgical site has not properly healed.

2. Patients with an ostomy should consider removing their ostomy appliance and adhesive. This will prevent extra radiation from treating that area of the skin. The skin around the ostomy and the stoma should be checked daily for problems.

3. Severe skin reactions are a reason to hold treatment to let the skin heal.

4. Topical lidocaine gel may soothe rectal discomfort.

5. Clothing considerations: avoid tight-fitting pants and underwear, which can cause friction and irritation. Women should also avoid wearing pantyhose and girdles. Loose cotton clothing and underwear are recommended for both men and women.

6. Patients should avoid chemical, mechanical, thermal, or other potential skin irritants.

❖ Fatigue

1. Fatigue is a significant problem for patients with CRC due to the large radiation field, concurrent chemotherapy, recent surgery, treatment-related nutritional deficits, and pain.

2. Fatigue is one of the most distressing side effects. It has a cumulative effect lasting throughout therapy. The patient's energy level gradually increases back to normal over

several months following completion of treatment.

❖ Myelosuppression

1. Approximately 15% to 25% of an adult's bone marrow is located in the pelvis.[12] Radiation therapy can deplete stem cells thereby affecting all blood cell lines, which can increase the patients risk of infection, bleeding, and anemia.

2. The degree of potential myelosuppression depends on the amount of pelvis in the radiation field and if the patient is receiving combined modality therapy.

❖ Diarrhea

1. The gastrointestinal tract (GI) is particularly sensitive to the effects of radiation due to the cells very short life span.

2. The timing and severity of diarrhea will be influenced the treatment plan, radiation therapy alone or in combination with chemotherapy.

3. Light exercise, i.e., walking, may help a patient move gas through the GI tract.

4. Patients with a history of irritable bowel syndrome or Crohn's disease should be followed closely for any exacerbation of symptoms induced by the therapy.

5. Hemorrhoids may also become inflamed and irritated; therefore, close attention should be paid to the anal area. The patient should

avoid any straining at stooling to prevent added pressure.

❖ Cystitis

1. Late cystitis leading to stricture of the bladder is a rare side effect. DMSO instillations may be helpful.

❖ Reproduction and sexual side effects

1. The impact of therapy on the patient with CRC should not be understated.

2. Effects on women: need for contraception measures during treatment to prevent pregnancy; the cervix and uterus may atrophy; there may vaginitis with or without pain as an early side effect or vaginal stenosis with painful intercourse as a late effect; premature menopause can occur in women with ovarian function and treatment with a hormone replacement therapy can be considered. Vaginal dilators or creams and exercises may be prescribed to prevent vaginal stenosis.

3. Effects on men: impotence may occur due to possible damage to nerves, blood vessels, and the testes.[13] There may also be a temporary decrease in sperm count, urethritis, and pain on ejaculation.

4. Both men and women should consider reproductive measures before starting therapy, i.e., sperm banking and egg harvesting. Referrals to counselors and/or therapists can be bene-

ficial. Alternative ways of expressing sexuality should be reviewed with the patient and significant other.

❖ Keys to effective symptom management

  ❖ Take all side effects seriously and treat them promptly
  ❖ Explain the cause of the side effects. Knowing what is expected versus unexpected can be empowering to patients.
  ❖ Educate the patient about when to call the radiation oncologist or nurse for questions and concerns. Note: the patient is in the treatment suite daily, and thus questions can often be addressed there.
  ❖ Provide clear explanations on self-care measures and symptom management strategies
  ❖ Be persistent in attempts to control symptoms. It is not a failure to keep trying strategies to manage a symptom until one is found that works.
  ❖ Remember to care for the whole person, physical and emotional

Additional Radiation Therapy Options

❖ Endocavitary radiation therapy

  ❖ Candidate: potentially curative early-stage rectal cancer with tumor size of ≤3 cm, more than 10cm above the anal verge, well- or moderately well-differentiated histology[3]

- ❖ Often performed in the radiation therapy department under local anesthetic
- ❖ Research supports its efficacy in local control and survival in carefully selected patients and may be used instead of surgery.[3]
- ❖ Procedure: Typically receives four 30 Gy treatments each separated by approximately 2 weeks[3]
- ❖ Side effects: acute—minor rectal bleeding in approximately 35%; rectal urgency in about 20%;[14] late effects include telangiectasia and mild fibrosis[12]

- ❖ Intraoperative radiation therapy (IORT)
  - ❖ IORT is delivered either with the use of a linear accelerator or the use of high dose rate (HDR) brachytherapy.
  - ❖ Indications: treat the exposed tumor bed or areas of unresectable gross tumor; boost dose in combination with large-field external beam radiation therapy and surgical resection[15]
  - ❖ IORT must be delivered in a specially designed room that is fully shielded for delivery of the radiation therapy. Other equipment is modified so the patient can be alone during the IORT portion of care, but still can be monitored.
  - ❖ Procedure:
    1. With the linear accelerator method, the patient has surgery then receives the radiation therapy. The linear accelerator is either built into the surgical suite or the patient

must be transported to the radiation therapy department.

2. With the HDR IORT method, the HDR machine is mobile; therefore, it can move between the surgical suite and the radiation therapy department. The applicator is securely placed onto the surgical bed, intraoperative shields are placed to protect surrounding tissue, and iridium-192 radioactive sources deliver the prescribed amount of radiation. The duration of treatment depends on the source of energy, number of fields, and total dose.[16]

3. After both methods, once the radiation has been delivered, the surgery is completed and the patient is taken to the recovery room.

* Side effects: peripheral nerve damage, infection/abscess, damage to ureter and/or blood vessel, delayed or impaired wound healing; fibrosis of the surgical anastomosis and/or fibrosis of the muscle, bone, or cartilage; and small bowel obstruction

* Hyperthermia[17]

  * Hyperthermia uses heat to treat cancer.
  * Currently it is being investigated in clinical trials to treat patients with rectal cancer.
  * It may be combined with external beam radiation therapy and/or chemotherapy and followed by surgery.

❖ Side effects: skin erythema, blistering, diarrhea, and local discomfort

References

1. Hilderly L. "Principles of Teletherapy." In Dow KH, Bucholtz JD, and Iwamoto RR, eds. *Nursing Care in Radiation Oncology*. Philadelphia, PA: WB Saunders Company, 1997: 6–20.

2. National Comprehensive Cancer Network (NCCN). "Colon and Rectal Cancer Treatment Guidelines." In *The Complete Library of Practice Guidelines in Oncology*, 2nd ed. Version 2001. Rockledge, PA: NCCN, 2001.

3. Martenson JA, and Gunderson LL. "Colon and Rectum." In Perez CA, and Brady LW, eds. *Principles and Practice of Radiation Oncology*. Philadelphia, PA: Lippincott-Raven, 1997: 1489–1510.

4. Minsky BD, Coia L, Haller DG, *et al.* "Radiation Therapy for Rectosigmoid and Rectal Cancer: Results of the 1992–1994 Patterns of Care Process Survey." *J Clin Oncol.* 1998; 16: 2542–2547.

5. Peeters M, and Haller DG. "Therapy for Early-Stage Colorectal Cancer." *Oncology.* 1999; 13: 307–315.

6. Minsky B. "Rectal Cancer." In Leibel SA, Phillips TL, eds. *Textbook of Radiation Oncology*, 3rd ed. Philadelphia, PA: WB Saunders Company, 1998: 686–702.

7. Minsky BD, Cohen AM, Kemeny N, *et al.* "Combined Modality Therapy of Rectal Cancer: Decreased Acute Toxicity with the Preoperative Approach." *J Clin Oncol.* 1992; 10: 1218–1224.

8. Minsky BD. "The Role of Adjuvant Radiation Therapy in the Treatment of Colorectal Cancer." *Hematol Oncol Clin North Am.* 1997; 11: 679–697.

9. Lewis WG, Williamson ME, Kuzu A, *et al.* "Potential Disadvantages of Post-operative Adjuvant

Radiotherapy After Anterior Resection for Rectal Cancer: A Pilot Study of Sphincter Function, Rectal Capacity and Clinical Outcome." *Int J Colorectal Dis.* 1995; 10: 133–137.

10. Minsky BD. "The Role of Radiation Therapy in Rectal Cancer." *Semin Oncol.* 1997; 24: S18-25–S18-29 (suppl 18).

11. Gosselin T. "Radiation Therapy." In Berg, D. ed. *Contemporary Issues in Colorectal Cancer: A Nursing Perspective.* Boston, MA: Jones and Bartlett Publishers, 2001: 135–156.

12. Hassey KM. "Radiation Therapy for Rectal Cancer and the Implications for Nursing." *Cancer Nurs.* 1987; 10: 311–318.

13. Witt ME, McDonald-Lynch A, and Grimmer D. "Adjuvant Radiotherapy to the Colorectum: Nursing Implications." *Oncol Nurs Forum.* 1987; 14: 17–21.

14. Chao KSC, Perez CA, Brady LW. Radiation Oncology: Management Decisions. Philadelphia, PA: Lippincott-Raven, 1999: 399–408.

15. Maher KE. "Principles of Radiation Therapy." In Nevidjon BM, and Sowers KW, eds. *A Nurse's Guide to Cancer Care.* Philadelphia, PA: Lippincott Williams & Wilkins, 2000: 215–240.

16. Wojtas F, Smith R. "Hyperthermia and Intraoperative Radiation Therapy." In Dow KH, ed. *Nursing Care in Radiation Oncology.* Philadelphia, PA: WB Saunders Company, 1997: 36–46.

17. Anscher MS, Lee C, Hurwitz H, *et al.* A Pilot Study of Preoperative Continuous Infusion 5-Fluorouracil, External Microwave Hyperthermia, and External Beam Radiotherapy for Treatment of Locally Advanced, Unresectable, or Recurrent Rectal Cancer. *Int J Radiat Oncol Biol Phys.* 2000; 47: 719–724.

9

Adjuvant Chemotherapy

Introduction

For most individuals with colorectal cancer (CRC), the curative treatment option is surgical resection of the primary tumor and regional lymph nodes. Despite this best practice, almost 50% of individuals initially treated in this manner will development recurrent disease.[1] The standard of care is to add adjuvant chemotherapy and/or radiotherapy for specific stages of disease. Guidelines from the National Comprehensive Cancer Network (NCCN) have been established to guide practitioners in treating patients with colon and rectal carcinomas. These guidelines serve as the basis for the recommendations outlined in this section.

Standard Adjuvant Chemotherapy: General Principles

❖ Definition: additional therapy given after potentially curative surgery

❖ Goal: eradicate any residual malignant cells before they develop into new tumors

❖ Surgical pathologic stage of the primary tumor is the most important prognostic tool and the one factor that dictates the need for adjuvant therapy.

Principles of Adjuvant Chemotherapy for Colon Cancer

❖ Therapeutic options are based on the stage of disease at the time of diagnosis.

❖ If patients are surgical candidates, they should also be candidates for adjuvant therapy, if it is warranted based on stage of disease.

  ❖ A patient's age alone should not be an exclusion for adjuvant therapy. Older age patients, i.e., those greater than 65 years at diagnosis benefit from therapy with acceptable toxicity.[2] These benefits have been the same as those seen in younger patients with the same characteristics.[2]

  ❖ Adjuvant therapy is considered cost effective (costing approximately $5000 per life year saved) and should be offered to all patients for specific stages of disease who have undergone surgery with curative intent.[3]

* Combination therapy has been shown to improve survival whereas single agent therapy is no better than postoperative observation.[1]

Treatment Recommendations

❖ Stage I colon cancer: treated with curative surgery only[4]

* Adjuvant therapy does not improve overall survival and is not recommended.

❖ Stage II colon cancer (no lymph node involvement): adjuvant therapy is controversial; if administered at this time, it is best instituted in the context of a well-designed clinical trial.[4]

* Most research does not show an improvement in survival for patients given adjuvant therapy compared to untreated patients.[5]
* Individuals whose cancer was perforated or obstructed, had positive tumor margins, and/or adhered to local organs are considered at high risk of recurrence and may be treated with adjuvant chemotherapy.[4]
* Additional tumor features that may delineate individuals at high risk are under investigation and include ploidy, *p*53 status, thymidylate synthesis levels, and chromosomal mutations.[5]

❖ Stage III colon cancer (lymph nodes are involved): the standard of care is adjuvant chemotherapy[4]

* In this patient population, adjuvant chemotherapy in addition to curative surgery has been the

standard treatment strategy since 1990.[6] It has reduced the risk of tumor recurrence by 41% to 50% and has prolonged overall survival.[4,5]

❖ If perforation is present at the time of diagnosis, the NCCN recommends adding radiation therapy to 5-FU and leucovorin (LV).[4]

Principles of Adjuvant Chemotherapy for Rectal Cancer

❖ Therapeutic options in rectal cancer are also based on the stage of disease at the time of diagnosis, but the patterns of treatment failure are also important.

　❖ The rectum lies below the peritoneal reflection, with an anatomically limited surgical field; thus, rectal cancer often recurs locally, and a local adjuvant treatment, i.e., radiation therapy is very important.

　❖ Colon cancer, on the other hand, has a wide anatomic surgical field and different primary blood supply system; therefore, the cancer recurs in distant sites, thus local therapies have limited value. A systemic strategy with chemo- and/or immunotherapy is more appropriate.

Treatment Recommendations

❖ Stage I (no lymph node involvement): no adjuvant therapy is recommended.[4]

❖ Stage II and III rectal cancer: adjuvant radiotherapy with or without chemotherapy is recommended.[4]

❖ The specifics of adjuvant treatment of rectal cancer and radiotherapy are discussed in Chapter 8.

Adjuvant Therapy Regimens in Colon Cancer

❖ The backbone of adjuvant systemic chemotherapy is the thymidylate synthase (TS) inhibitor 5-fluorouracil (5-FU). The main adjuvant regimens incorporate 5-FU plus leucovorin (LV) or levamisole. The common regimens are noted in Table 9-1.

❖ Adjuvant 5-FU plus levamisole

  ❖ In 1990, this combination became the standard chemotherapeutic regimen in the adjuvant setting for stage III colon cancer.[6,7]

  ❖ Recently, the benefit of levamisole in this regimen has come into question, and though it is still an option, the NCCN does not currently recommend it.[4]

  ❖ Toxicities of the regimen include myelosuppression; elevations in liver enzymes; alterations in taste, including a metallic taste; general body aches; neurotoxicity; and depression. Because these side effects were often mild, they did not require discontinuation of therapy.[3]

TABLE 9-1
Common Adjuvant Chemotherapy Regimens[1,5]

Drug/Combination	Dose and Schedule
5-fluorouracil (5-FU) plus levamisole	
5-FU	450 mg/m2 IV days 1–5, then once weekly beginning day 28
Levamisole	50 mg every 8 hours PO on days 1–3, every other week
Treatment continues for 1 year	
5-fluorouracil (5-FU) plus low-dose leucovorin (Mayo)	
5-FU	425 mg/m2 IVP days 1–5 for two 4-week cycles, then every 5 weeks
Leucovorin (LV)	20 mg/m2 IVB days 1–5 for two 4-week cycles, then every 5 weeks immediately before 5-FU administration
Treatment continues for 6 months	
5-fluorouracil (5-FU) plus high-dose leucovorin (Roswell Park)	
5-FU	500 mg/m2 IVP (1 hour after start of LV) weekly for 6 weeks, every 8 weeks
Leucovorin (LV)	500 mg/m2 IV over 2 hours weekly for 6 weeks, every 8 weeks.
Treatment continues for 6 cycles	
Combination Chemotherapy/Radiation Therapy.[5]	
5-fluorouracil (5-FU) during radiation therapy	
5-FU	225 mg/m2/day continuous intravenous infusion during duration of radiation therapy
Radiation	180cGy Monday–Friday for a total of 25 doses to a total of 4,500 cGy, plus a boost dose of 180 cGy over 3 fractions. Overall total 5,040 cGy over 5–6 weeks.
5-fluorouracil (5-FU)–before and after radiation therapy	
5-FU	500 mg/m2/day IVP on days 1–5 monthly for 2 cycles both before and after radiation therapy.

❖ Adjuvant 5-FU and leucovorin (LV)

 ❖ There are two common regimens of 5-FU and LV, as illustrated in Table 9-1.

 ❖ This combination has shown significant improvement in disease-free survival and overall survival as compared with surgery alone.[3]

 ❖ Recent research has reported that 5-FU plus LV (given at low or high does) is at least as effective, and can be given in half the time, as 5-FU and levamisole; therefore, it has largely replaced the previous standard regimen.[1,5]

 ❖ Toxicities differ between the various 5-FU and LV regimens.[3]

   1. 5-FU plus low dose LV (Mayo regimen) commonly produces stomatitis and leukopenia.

   2. 5-FU plus high dose LV (Roswell Park [RPCI] regimen) commonly produces diarrhea.

   3. Women and patients over the age of 70 experience more stomatitis and leukopenia regardless of the regimen.[3]

 ❖ For patients with stage II disease and risk factors associated with an increased chance of recurrence, as noted previously, 5-FU and LV either with or without radiation therapy may be administered.[4]

❖ Other adjuvant regimens, such as methyl-CCNU, vincristine, and 5-FU (MOF); 5-FU, LV, and interferon; 5-FU, leucovorin, and levamisole; portal vein infusion of 5-FU; and continuous infusion of

5-FU plus levamisole have all been investigated in clinical trials and are not superior to the 5-FU plus LV regimens.[5]

Emerging Directions in Adjuvant Therapy in Colon Cancer

❖ Immunologic adjuvant therapy

- ❖ Prior attempts to use the patient's own immune system to destroy CRC cells have been unsuccessful, though this continues to be an area of great interest.
- ❖ Interferon-alfa, interleukin-2, and bacillus Calmette–Guerin (BCG) are not considered active immunotherapeutic agents in CRC.
- ❖ Edrecolomab (Panorex, Mab 17-1A) is a murine monoclonal antibody that binds to the 17-1A antigen. This antigen is prevalent on the majority of adenocarincomas, including CRC. A European trial reported that the adjuvant administration of edrecolomab increased disease-free and overall survival in patients with stage III colon cancer.[8] Clinical trials in the United States are closed to accrual and data analysis is pending. Known toxicities include infusion-related hypersensitivity, anaphylaxis, low-grade fever, abdominal pain, flulike symptoms, nausea, vomiting, and diarrhea.[9]

Promising New Research for Adjuvant Chemotherapy

❖ Clinical trials completed to accrual but awaiting results

❖ The National Surgical Bowel and Breast Project (NSABP) compared UFT (uracil plus tegafur [Orzel]) to 5-FU and LV. This trial is interesting because it compares an oral agent (UFT) with the standard intravenous agents.

❖ The Cancer and Leukemia Group B led an international effort comparing standard weekly 5-FU and LV either alone or in combination with irinotecan. In addition, this trial had two correlative science questions. One study was prospectively assessing several cellular features (e.g., TS, *p53*, vascular endothelial growth factor [VEGF], the deleted-in-colon-cancer (*DCC*) gene, microsatellite instability [MSI], and topoisomerase I levels) on recurrence and survival. The second study was looking at the influence of diet and physical activity on toxicity, recurrence, and survival.[10]

❖ Roche Oncology sponsored two trials of the same design comparing 5-FU plus low-dose LV to capecitabine in patients with stage II and III colon cancer. Additional comparisons on quality of life, health economics, and molecular features, such as thymidylate synthesis [TS], thymidine phosphorylase [TP], and dihydropyrimidine dehydrogenase [DPD] levels on tumor response are being analyzed.[10]

❖ European investigators favor continuous infusion administration of 5-FU; therefore, their adjuvant clinical trials have compared infusional 5-FU and LV either alone or in combination with irinotecan and infusional 5-FU and LV either alone or in combination with oxaliplatin. The later study included both patients with stage II and III disease.[10]

❖ Once the data is available, these clinical trials will define the adjuvant chemotherapy offered to future U.S. patients with stage II and III colon cancer. In addition, the analyzes on prognostic tumor markers, pathologic cellular features, and lifestyle habits and any impact they may have on recurrence and survival may provide valuable information that could assist clinicians in "tailoring" therapy to an individual's cancer.

❖ Ongoing U.S. clinical trials open to accrual

  ❖ The NSABP is randomizing patients with either stage II or III colon cancer to standard weekly 5-FU and LV with or without oxaliplatin.[10]

  ❖ A European study in stage II colon cancer is comparing surgery to 5-FU, LV, and irinotecan chemotherapy.

  ❖ Another European trial is looking at the role of cyclooxygenase inhibitors in adjuvant therapy. In this trial, investigators will give patients an adjuvant chemotherapy regimen of their choice. Then the patients will be randomized to receive

one of four treatments: placebo for 2 or 5 years
or rolecoxib 25 mg/day for 2 or 5 years.[11]

❖ Many of the recent U.S. clinical trials have just
recently closed; therefore, there are only
proposed concepts at this time.

Adjuvant Therapy in Rectal Cancer

❖ Since the 1990s, combined chemotherapy and
pelvic radiation therapy has been recommended
for patients with stage II and III rectal cancer.[6]

  ❖ The current approach is 5-FU for 2 months
  prior to and after radiation therapy, radiation (a
  total of 4,500 to 5,040 cGY) plus continuous-
  infusion 5-FU during radiation over approximately 5 to 6 weeks.[1]

Promising New Research for Adjuvant Therapy in Rectal Cancer

❖ The Radiation Therapy Oncology Group (RTOG) is
looking at preoperative combined modality therapy.

  ❖ The trial will compare radiotherapy given twice
  a day, Monday through Friday for 19 days plus
  continuous infusion 5-FU compared to daily
  doses of radiation therapy plus continuous
  infusion 5-FU both given on Monday through
  Friday for 25 days and irinotecan given on day
  1 of each week for 4 weeks. Within 4 to 10
  weeks all patients will have surgery.[10]

❖ Investigations of less invasive surgical procedures
are also under way.

Follow-up Recommendations for Colorectal Cancer

❖ Primary treatment ends and follow-up care begins.[12]

  ❖ The American Society of Clinical Oncology (ASCO) recommends a range of procedures and tests as part of the medical care for individuals after treatment for CRC.[12]

    1. Physical examination every 3 to 6 months for 3 years, then yearly
    2. Colonoscopy within the first year after primary treatment; if negative repeat every 3 to 5 years
    3. Carcinoembryonic antigen (CEA) every 2 to 3 months for 2 years, then at the physician's discretion
    4. Liver function tests, fecal occult blood test, complete blood test, computed tomography (CT) scan, and chest x-ray are not recommended as a regular follow up. These tests may be in order if there are suspicious signs or symptoms.
    5. Lipid-associated sialic acid (LASA), CA 19-9, DNA ploidy, *p*53, and *ras* are experimental tumor markers and are not recommended, outside the context of a clinical trial, as part of regular follow-up.
    6. In addition, patients with stage II or III rectal cancer who have not been treated with radi-

ation therapy should have a proctosigmoidoscopy every 6 to 12 months.[12]

Nursing Implications of Adjuvant Chemotherapy

❖ Nurses are essential to helping patients maintain their quality of life while receiving adjuvant chemotherapy by:

 ❖ Educating the patient and significant others about the disease, treatment plans, and expected side effects
 ❖ Helping patients understand their treatment options through participating in the shared decision-making process
 ❖ Providing written information to reinforce educational information; materials must take into consideration the patient's literacy level, spoken language, and cultural background.
 ❖ Proactively recommending measures for symptom prevention and management
 ❖ Assessing the patient thoroughly at baseline and at regular intervals during therapy to determine response to symptom management measures
 ❖ Coordinating patient care, especially in multimodality treatment regimens
 ❖ Providing emotional support to patients and significant others in the form of one-to-one discussions or support groups

❖ Most patients tolerate adjuvant therapy for carcinomas of the colon and rectum quite well.

❖ Some, but not all patients, need to make lifestyle modifications, e.g., changing from working full time to part time, during therapy.

❖ Common toxicities with adjuvant 5-FU-base regimens

  ❖ Stomatitis
  ❖ Leukopenia
  ❖ Diarrhea
  ❖ Skin changes: increased sensitivity to the sun; hyperpigmentation
  ❖ Less common and often mild and temporary side effects, which will not be discussed here, are nausea, vomiting, hair loss, changes in nails, cerebellar ataxia, increased tearing, conjunctivitis, blurred vision, and photophobia.

❖ Nursing care measures are outline in Table 9-2.

❖ The National Cancer Institute (NCI) Common Toxicity Criteria (CTC) is invaluable at providing a common language to evaluate and describe toxicities. The criteria for the most common toxicities are illustrated in Appendix A.

TABLE 9-2

Potential Adjuvant Therapy–Induced Side Effects and Suggested Interventions

Side Effect	Average Onset	Interventions	Comments
Stomatitis	Approximately 5–8 days after start of therapy	Gently cleansing of the mouth at least twice a day and after meals; assess mucosa prior to and during therapy—report changes. Maintain good nutrition. Avoid foods and beverages that are irritating or that will potentially burn the mucosa. For severe stomatitis, antibacterial and/or antifungal rinses may be suggested. Topical or systemic pain medications may help with discomfort.	May be severe in some cases. Moderate or severe stomatitis would be a reason to delay therapy until it has resolved. Dose modifications in subsequent doses/cycles may be considered.

(continued)

TABLE 9-2
Potential Adjuvant Therapy–Induced Side Effects and Suggested Interventions (continued)

Side Effect	Average Onset	Interventions	Comments
Neutropenia associated with leukopenia	Approximately 10–14 days after start of therapy	Monitor blood counts; monitor temperature at least twice a day. Avoid exposure to possible infections. Infection precautions.	May be enhanced when combined with leucovorin. Severe leukopenia would be a reason to delay therapy. Dose modifications in subsequent doses/cycles may be considered.
Diarrhea	Approximately 7–14 days after start of therapy	Take antidiarrheal medications as prescribed. Drink 8–10 glasses of fluids each day. Eat a low-residue, low lactose diet. Monitor bowel habits and report any changes.	May be enhanced when combined with leucovorin. Moderate or severe diarrhea is a reason to delay therapy until it has resolved. Dose modifications in subsequent doses/cycles may be considered.
Skin reactions: Sensitivity to sun Hyperpigmentation of skin	Varies, but usually after several cycles of therapy	Avoid exposure to the skin, wear hats, and cover exposed arms and legs; wear sunscreen year-round. Rotate veins used for 5-FU administration or use a central venous access device.	May negatively impact self-image.

References

1. Ellenhorn JDI, Coia LR, Alberts SR, and Hoff PM. "Colorectal and Anal Cancers." In Pazdur R, Coia LR, Hoskins HJ, and Wagman LD, eds. *Cancer Management: A Multidisciplinary Approach*, 6th ed. Melville, NY: PRR, Inc, 2002: 295–318.

2. Sargent D, Goldberg R, MacDonald J, *et al.* "Adjuvant Chemotherapy for Colon Cancer Is Beneficial Without Significantly Increased Toxicity in Elderly Patients: Results from 3351 Patient Meta-analysis." *Proc Am Soc Clin Oncol.* 2000; 19: 933 (abstr).

3. MacDonald JS. "Adjuvant Therapy of Colon Cancer." *CA: Cancer J Clin.* 1999; 49(4): 202–219.

4. National Comprehensive Cancer Network (NCCN). "Colon and Rectal Cancer Treatment Guidelines." In *The Complete Library of Practice Guidelines in Oncology*, 2nd ed. Version 2001. Rockledge, PA: NCCN; 2001.

5. Goldberg RM. "Gastrointestinal Tract Cancers." In Casciato DA, and Lowitz BB, eds. *Manual of Clinical Oncology.* 4th ed. Philadelphia, PA: Lippincott Williams & Wilkins, 2000: 182–194.

6. National Institutes of Health consensus conference. "Adjuvant Therapy for Patients with Colon and Rectal Cancer." *JAMA.* 1990; 264(11): 1444–1450.

7. Moertel CG, Fleminng TR, MacDonald JS, *et al.* "Fluorouracil Plus Levamisole as Effective Adjuvant Therapy After Resection of Stage III Colon Carcinoma: A Final Report." *Ann Intern Med.* 1995; 122: 321–326.

8. Riethmüller G, Holz E, Schlimok G, *et al.* "Monoclonal Antibody Therapy for Resected Dukes' C Colorectal Cancer: Seven-Year Outcome of a Multicenter Randomized Trial." *J Clin Oncol.* 1998; 16: 1788–1794.

9. Fields LA, Nagy A, Schwartzberg L, *et al.* "Edrecolomab (Panorex, 17-1a Antibody) Alone or in Combination with 5-FU Based Chemotherapy in Adjuvant Treatment of Stage III Colon Cancer: A Safety Review." *Proc Am Soc Clin Oncol.* 1999; 18: 1676 (abstr).

10. National Cancer Institute Cancer Clinical Trials. Available at http://cancer.gov. Accessed June 30, 2002.

11. Haller, DG. "Colorectal Cancer Treatment of Advanced Disease and Adjuvant Therapy." May 20. 2002. Available at http://virtualmeeting.asco.org/vm2002/gastro.cfm. Accessed June 30, 2002.

12. American Society of Clinical Oncology (ASCO). *A Patient's Guide: Follow Up Care for Colorectal Cancer.* Alexandria, VA: ASCO, 2001.

PART IV

Treatment of Recurrent and Metastatic Colorectal Cancer

10

Regional Treatment Approaches: Focus on Hepatic Disease

Introduction

Of the more than 130,000 people who develop colorectal cancer (CRC) each year, half will develop a recurrence at some point in their lifetime.[1] The liver is the most common site of metastasis. Surgery with or without systemic chemotherapy as well as intralesion strategies are often utilized as treatment methods.

Anatomy, Physiology, and the Pathophysiology of Liver Metastasis

❖ The liver has two main anatomic lobes (right and left), which are subdivided into caudate and quadrate lobes. The right hepatic lobe is divided into four segments, while the left lobe is divided into two segments.[2]

❖ There are two sources of blood supply to the liver—the hepatic artery and the hepatic portal vein. It is the hepatic portal vein that brings materials from the digestive tract to the liver.

❖ The liver is the first visceral organ that cancer cells of gastrointestinal origin encounter after release into capillaries, venules, and finally, the portal circulation.[3]

Considerations Relating to the Treatment of Metastases

❖ Extent of hepatic involvement is an important predictor of survival.[4]

  ◆ Untreated patients with liver-only disease replacing more than 50% of normal liver rarely survived more than 2 years.

  ◆ Of those patients with untreated solitary metastasis, more than 20% survive at least 3 years; length of survival and the number of lesions are inversely correlated; 24 months for those with three or fewer lesions, and 10 months for those with four or more lesions.[5] An inverse correlation is also noted between survival and number of involved lobes; 21 months for those with solitary unilobar metastasis, and 15 months for patients with multiple liver lesions.

❖ Patients untreated with extrahepatic disease survive a median of 9 months compared to 18 months for those with liver-only disease.[6]

❖ A recent report suggests that selected patients with both hepatic and pulmonary metastases from CRC can benefit from resections. Those having their first metastasis confined to the liver had a longer survival than those who presented with isolated lung disease or disease in both the lung and liver. The median survival once a patient had both liver and lung metastases resected was 3.8 years.[7]

Current Treatment Options for Metastasis

- ❖ Surgical resection with or without pre- and/or postoperative chemotherapy

- ❖ Hepatic Arterial Infusion (HAI)

- ❖ Radiofrequency Ablation (RFA)

- ❖ Selective Internal Radiation Therapy

- ❖ Ethanol or Acetic Acid Injections

- ❖ Chemoembolization

- ❖ Cryosurgery

Surgical Resection of Metastatic Liver Lesions

- ❖ Recommended treatment if lesion(s) are isolated to the liver and localized within the lobes. Still considered the "gold" standard approach. See Figure 10-1.

- ❖ Approximately 10% of patients who develop liver metastasis are eligible for curative resection.[6]

- ❖ Up to 75% of the liver can be surgically removed, because it can regenerate.[6]

FIGURE 10-1
Common liver resections for metastatic colorectal cancer: **A:** Right lobectomy. **B:** Left lobectomy. **C:** Right trisegmentectomy. **D:** Left lateral segmentectomy. **E:** Left triseg-mentectomy.

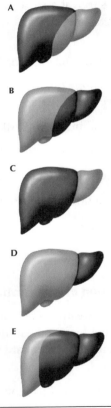

Source: Saddler DA, and Lassere Y. "Management of Hepatic Disease." In Berg DT, ed. *Contemporary Issues in Colorectal Cancer: A Nursing Perspective.* Boston, MA: Jones and Bartlett Publishers; 2001; 203–221. Reprinted with permission.

❖ Combination therapy is often at least considered, e.g., RFA, HAI, or systemic chemotherapy; therapy may be given neoadjuvantly to reduce tumor bulk and thereby convert the patient to a surgical candidate, or adjuvantly to reduce tumor recurrence.

❖ Postoperatively patients remain in the hospital for 2 or more weeks, and require an additional 1 to 2 months of recovery time before resuming routine activities.[6]

❖ Efficacy

  ❖ Approximately half of the patients after resection suffer a recurrence, 25% are alive without disease at 5 years, and 33% are alive (with or without disease) at 5 years.[8]

  ❖ Morbidity and mortality rates are low and long-term side effects seldom occur.[8]

Patient Selection

❖ Perioperative risk, technical feasibility and respectability of the liver lesions, and evaluation for long-term survival are key considerations.

❖ Comorbid disease should not shorten lifespan to time point less than the cancer; cirrhosis, hepatitis B or C, and chronic alcohol abuse must be considered.

❖ Contraindications (due to lack of long-term survival benefit):[6]

  ❖ Portal lymph node metastases
  ❖ Coexistent extrahepatic recurrence

- ❖ The presence of four or more liver metastases
- ❖ Inability to preserve an adequate volume of functional hepatic parenchyma (require at least 20% normal hepatic parenchyma after resection)
- ❖ Inability to obtain at least a 1-cm tumor-free margin. *Note:* 5-year survival rate is 60% for patients with at least a 1-cm tumor-free margin; 30% for those with less than a 1-cm tumor-free margin; and no survivors when the surgical margins are positive.[9]
- ❖ Hepatic vein confluence/inferior vena cava involvement by tumor
- ❖ Main portal vein bifurcation involvement by tumor

Preoperative Workup

- ❖ Computed tomography (CT) portography defines the extent of intrahepatic disease.

- ❖ Chest x-ray is usually sufficient to assess the lungs unless an abnormality is noted, then a chest CT or a biopsy is indicated.

- ❖ Positron emission tomography (PET) scans, magnetic resonance imaging (MRI), and/or biopsy evaluate the abdomen and pelvis for potential sites of recurrence.

- ❖ Colonoscopy is indicated, if the disease-free interval has been more than 2 years and if one has not been done previously.

❖ Intraoperative ultrasonography (IOUS) of the liver is used to identify intrahepatic course of the hepatic veins, discover small tumors not detected on preoperative CT scans, and/or ascertain involvement of key vascular structures, preventing tumor free margins.

❖ Preoperative angiography is usually not required for anatomic definition unless a hepatic artery infusion pump is being considered.

Surgical Procedure

❖ Three components are involved—determination of resectability, inflow and outflow vascular control, and dissection of the liver parenchyma.

❖ An adequate manual and visual exploration of the abdomen, pelvis, liver, and lymph node areas is important to assess for other sites of recurrence.

❖ The actual surgical technique, e.g., a segmental or wedge resection requires expertise on behalf of the surgeon and frequent use of the IOUS.

❖ The cut edge of the liver parenchyma is extensively coagulated. Closed suction drains are placed around the operative site to collect any residual blood or bile that may accumulate in the immediate postoperative period.

Postoperative Nursing Implications[6]

❖ First 24 hours are critical

❖ Nurses must know what complications to anticipate, signs of impending problems, and how to
manage problems as they arise.[6]

❖ Care focuses on intravascular volume management and prevention of pulmonary complications.

❖ Surgical drains are removed within 48 to 72 hours
in the absence of a biliary leak.

❖ Frequent assessment of vital signs, abdominal
girth, surgical incision for successful healing and
to rule out infection, and patency of drains are
very important and should help prevent life-
threatening situations.[6]

❖ Potential complications:[6] hemorrhage, biliary
leak, biloma, subphrenic abscess, infection, pneumonia, pleural effusion, transient metabolic consequences, portal hypertension, portal vein
thrombosis, clotting defects, ileus, hepatic failure,
hypotension, tachycardia, and increasing abdominal girth[6]

1. Hemorrhage: possible signs include hypotension, tachycardia, increased abdominal girth,
   and a decrease in the hemoglobin and hematocrit.

2. Postoperative ileus is usually short-term; medications, fluids, and nutrition can be restarted
   within 48 hours.

3. Pneumonia and pleural effusion are common
   problems, but are usually asymptomatic and

do not require drainage. Aggressive pulmonary toilet, with deep breathing and coughing, and incentive spirometry are required.

4. Ascites may occur after the drainage tubes are removed. Sodium restriction of 1,000 to 1,500 mg/day, fluid restriction of 1,500 mL per day, loop diuretic, and spironolactone are often helpful.[2]

5. Elevated liver function enzymes may represent vascular inflow or outflow injury, hepatic failure, portal vein thrombosis and/or obstruction. A Doppler ultrasound can be a helpful diagnostic tool.

6. Biloma (collection of bile): pain, fever, and distended abdomen are common symptoms.

7. Perihepatic infection or necrosis of the remaining liver may result in a subphrenic abscess. Signs and symptoms would include sharp right upper quadrant pain and low-grade fever.

8. Bleeding should be reported to the surgeon immediately. Transfusions with fresh-frozen plasma may be required.

9. Alterations in mental status and increased ammonia levels may be seen in the face of impending liver failure.

❖ Laboratory assessments:

  ❖ Hemoglobin and hematocrit: decrease may signal hemorrhage.

- Liver function tests (LFTs): generally rise initially postoperatively, but should decrease to normal within a week or so.
- Serum glucose—abnormalities may cause hepatic failure.[6]
- Electrolytes and creatinine should be monitored closely. Replace electrolytes as needed.[2]
- Coagulation studies
- Urine and stool output—abnormalities may signal hemorrhage or other problems.

Chemotherapy

- Fewer than 5% of patients with metastases have disease confirmed only to the liver; therefore, chemotherapy may be the primary treatment or added to the therapeutic plan.[10]

- Chemotherapy may be given pre- or postoperatively.

  - Patients who have an objective response to preoperative chemotherapy also have a significant improvement in disease-free survival.[10] Patients who do not respond to the chemotherapy have a shorter disease-free survival.
  - Preoperative chemotherapy is given to reduce the tumor size and to ensure tumor-free resection margins.
  - No survival benefit has been demonstrated with the neoadjuvant administration of fluorouracil, oxaliplatin, and folinic acid.[2]

Second Hepatectomy

❖ Of those patients who do recur after initial surgery, approximately 50% to 60% recur within the liver. Repeat hepatectomy is possible, because the liver regenerates to its approximate original size within 4 to 6 weeks.[6]

❖ Repeat resection on metastases is technically more challenging due to adhesions, changes in the shape of the organ, and vascular structures subsequent to regeneration.

❖ Operative mortality and morbidity rates are similar to initial resection.

❖ The factors most important when considering a second resection are the patient's overall medical health, the number of lesions, and the size of the largest lesions. Patients who have small, solitary tumors, which can be easily removed, should be selected for repeat resection.[11]

Hepatic Arterial Infusion (HAI) Chemotherapy

❖ HAI provides a higher concentration of chemotherapy to the liver lesions than could be achieved through systemic administration. Normal liver tissue receives significantly less drug. This is achievable as a consequence of the dual blood supply provided by the portal vein and hepatic artery.[1,12]

❖ May be given as adjuvant therapy following hepatic resection for metastases or as treatment for unresectable liver metastases.

❖ Efficacy: Response rates range from 30% to 50% in patients previously treated, which is higher than most systemic chemotherapy regimens, but HAI has not been shown to impact survival.[12] Research is ongoing in this area. In one single-institution study, 2-year survival and hepatic disease-free survival were improved by 14% and 30% respectively with adjuvant HAI plus systemic chemotherapy after hepatic resection compared to postoperative systemic chemotherapy alone.[13] Five-year survival was not different. In a second study coordinated by a cooperative group, despite improvements in hepatic disease-free survival, there was no difference in overall survival.[14]

❖ The role of HAI therapy as an adjuvant treatment after liver resection is still undefined.[1]

Patient Selection

❖ In the adjuvant setting for patients with resected liver metastases

❖ For patients with unresectable hepatic metastases, patients who have failed systemic therapy for metastatic CRC, or who have an intolerance to systemic therapy

Preoperative Workup

❖ Assess surgical and medical fitness

❖ Angiography, with selective injection of the celiac and superior mesenteric arteries, should be done before the hepatic pump is placed to determine anatomic definition.

  ❖ Normal anatomy consists of the common hepatic artery arising from the celiac artery. The common hepatic artery separates into the right and left hepatic arteries.[15]

  ❖ Variant anatomy may be noted and includes the common hepatic artery dividing into three branches, a replaced right or left hepatic artery, or the common hepatic artery arising from the superior mesenteric artery.[15]

Surgical Procedure

❖ Several specialists are involved in the successful implantation of HAI pumps such as the surgeon, invasive radiologist, operating room staff, and nuclear medicine radiologist.[1]

❖ An exploratory laparotomy is performed first to determine if extrahepatic metastases are present.

  ❖ If extrahepatic metastases are located and confirmed, placement of the HAI pump is contraindicated.[1]

  ❖ If there are no extrahepatic metastases, the pump can be placed.

❖ The implantable pump is placed in a subcutaneous fatty pocket, in an area above the incision, on the lower abdominal wall. A thin flap is placed over the pump, allowing for palpation and access to the pump diaphragm.

❖ The pump is positioned within the pocket so that the bolus access port is between the 3 and 6 o'clock positions.

❖ To avoid hematoma formation and to decrease infection, complete hemostatis in the pocket is essential.

❖ After the pump is sutured in place in the pocket, the catheter is placed into the hepatic artery, brought through the fascia and the peritoneum, and connected to the pump.[1] A fluorescein solution is injected through the pump bolus access port or the port chamber and monitored with an ultraviolet light to determine adequate perfusion of both lobes of the liver, as well as any misperfusion.

❖ A cholecystectomy is often performed at the time of pump placement.

❖ A nuclear scan is used to assess pump perfusion, as extrahepatic perfusion must be ruled out and bilobular flow must be documented before the surgery is completed.

HAI Procedure

❖ Floxuridine (FUDR) or 5-fluorouracil with or without leucovorin are the common agents delivered by HAI. The drugs are injected into the port chamber every two weeks alternating with equal cycles of heparinized saline. Dexamethasone may be added to the chemotherapy regimen to decrease biliary toxicity.[12]

❖ Systemic chemotherapy with many of the currently available agents may also be administered (see Chapter 11).

Postoperative Nursing Implications

❖ Potential complications:
  ❖ Partial or complete thrombosis of the hepatic artery
  ❖ Leakage of infusion solution from the artery
  ❖ Gastroduodenal irritation and/or ulceration
  ❖ Inadequate liver perfusion
  ❖ Chemical hepatitis
  ❖ Acalculous cholecystitis
  ❖ Sclerosing cholangitis
  ❖ Occlusion or displacement of the catheter
  ❖ Bile duct strictures and/or obstruction

Nursing Implications of the HAI Method of Chemotherapy Administration

❖ Actual drug administration—refilling of the pump chamber with prescribed chemotherapy and heparin solution—may be a nursing function.

❖ Knowledge of potential adverse events, such as gastritis, duodenitis, bleeding, infection, pump inversion, malfunction, clotting, disconnection, perforation, extravasations, dislodgement, or perfusion problems, in addition to those listed previously. Note: side effects may vary if systemic chemotherapy is also being administered and by what chemotherapy agents are in the regimen.

❖ Recommendations for symptom strategies, i.e., prophylactic therapies such as H_2 blockers to prevent gastroduodenal irritation and gastric ulcers[6]

❖ Patient education—Topics include:
  ❖ Rationale and logistics of the treatment
  ❖ Potential side effects and self-care measures
  ❖ Situations that may alter pump flow rates, such as exercise, saunas, any temperature changes, and changes in altitude
  ❖ The information card about the pump should be carried with the patient at all times, in case needed in locations with metal detection devices, i.e., airports and federal buildings, and if medical care is required while away from home.

❖ Pumps often remain in place even when no longer in use, but they can be removed electively or emergently.

Targeted Intralesion Therapy

❖ Intralesion therapies, such as ethanol injections, percutaneous acetic acid injections, radiofrequency ablation, chemoembolization, and cryotherapy may be used alone or in combination with other forms of treatment. Most of these therapies are under investigation.

❖ Candidates are those with small discrete lesions and no extrahepatic disease.

Nursing Implications for Intralesion Therapy

❖ Primary role—education and support regarding the procedure, potential side effects, and symptom assessment

Radiofrequency Ablation (RFA)

❖ Candidates:
  ❖ Appropriate for patients with unresectable liver metastases; lesions should be distinct, no larger than 5 cm, and no more than 4 in number.[16]
  ❖ May be contraindicated in patients with lesions close to large blood vessels, impaired coagulation (partial thromboplastin [PT] greater than 50%), thrombocytopenia (platelet count less than 50,000/µL).[16]

  ❖ Investigation as a treatment for pulmonary
    lesions is ongoing.[17]

❖ Preprocedure considerations:

  ❖ Full medical and laboratory assessment, including
    alpha-fetoprotein and carcinoembryonic antigen
  ❖ Staging by at least liver ultrasound, abdominal
    spiral CT scan, magnetic resonance imaging
    (MRI), chest x-ray, and bone scintigraphy[15]
  ❖ Preoperative teaching includes bowel prep, pul-
    monary toilet, pain management, wound care,
    and postoperative ambulation.

❖ Performed either percutaneously, laparoscopically,
  or during an open laparotomy. Anesthesia may be
  local, conscious, or general depending on the
  selected procedure.

❖ RFA technique uses expandable electrode needles
  to heat the tumor tissue plus a tumor-free margin.
  Frictional heating to temperatures exceeding 60°C
  causes a direct coagulation necrosis resulting in
  cell death. The procedure takes 6 to 12 minutes
  for each needle insertion.[16]

❖ Immediate complications may include bleeding at
  the needle insertion site, low-grade fever (lasting
  up to 3 days), malaise, slight elevation in
  transaminase levels, and/or thermal damage to
  adjacent organs. Infection, pneumothorax, skin
  burn, cardiac arrhythmia, and pleural effusions
  are not common but are possible.[16]

❖ The patient generally remains in the hospital for 24 hours, during which time liver and renal functions are monitored.

❖ Effectiveness, as evaluated by CT scans to identify any opacified foci representative of tumor necrosis, is in the range of 66% to 77% with approximately 68% of lesions showing no evidence of tumor progression after 6 months.[16]

❖ May be given in collaboration with chemotherapy; if so, RFA should be given two weeks prior to or after chemotherapy. The efficacy of this approach is still under investigation.[6]

Ethanol Injections and Percutaneous Acetic Acid Injections

❖ The administration of absolute ethanol into hepatic lesions may be done by percutaneous injection or during surgery. The alcohol causes cell death by dehydrating the tumor cells.

❖ Percutaneous acetic acid injection works by dissolving lipids and extracting collagen to cause cell death of the tumor cells.[6]

❖ The effectiveness of these procedures is questionable.

❖ Contraindications:[6]
  ❖ Large tumors, i.e., greater than 3 to 4 cms
  ❖ Partial thromboplastin (PT) less than 40%
  ❖ Platelet count less than 40,000/μL
  ❖ Advanced cirrhosis

❖ Extrahepatic disease

❖ Thrombosis of the main vein or portal branches

❖ Biliary tree dilation

❖ Possible complications:[6]

  ❖ Pain during injection. Helpful to keep the needle in place for up to 30 seconds then remove it slowly.

  ❖ Alcohol intoxication, especially if large volumes of alcohol are injected[2]

  ❖ Abnormal liver function enzymes due to hepatic necrosis, hemolysis, and localized thrombosis

Chemoembolization

❖ Like HAI, chemoembolization utilizes the hepatic artery to treat the metastatic lesions with high concentrations of chemotherapy.[6]

❖ This technique administers a mixture of a foreign substance, which stops the hepatic blood flow leading to the metastatic lesions, and chemotherapy. The chemotherapy agents commonly used include doxorubicin and cisplatin.

❖ A catheter is inserted in the femoral artery and fed up to the hepatic artery. Once in place, the mixture is injected.

❖ Cells die to due hypoxia from lack of blood flow and cytotoxicity of the chemotherapy agent.

❖ Side effects commonly include abdominal pain, nausea, vomiting, fever, fatigue, and potential liver failure.

❖ The efficacy of this technique is debatable. It has not yet shown a survival advantage.

Cryosurgery (Cryotherapy)

❖ It involves direct freezing of lesions, resulting in coagulation necrosis.

❖ Five-year survival rates of approximately 22% have been reported with this procedure.[6]

❖ Procedure:

   ❖ Performed via an exploratory laparotomy to first explore the abdomen to exclude extrahepatic disease and nodal deposits. The liver is then fully assessed both by intraoperative ultrasound (IOUS) and by the surgeon visually. Using IOUS, the cryoprobe is placed into the tumor. One or more probes are inserted into the lesion as needed based on its size. Each lesion is frozen for 15 minutes, thawed for 10 minutes, and then frozen again for another 15 minutes. At the end of the procedure, homeostasis is checked and the wound closed. Suction drains may be placed above and below the liver.[6]

   ❖ Possible complications: death, hypothermia, biliary fistulas, bleeding, thrombocytopenia, liver surface cracking fracture, consumptive coagulopathy, cryogenic shock, iatrogenic cryoprobe injuries, electrolyte disturbances, nitrogen embolism, intrahepatic abscess, subphrenic abscess, pleural effusions, acute renal failure, acute tubular necrosis, myoglobinuria, transient elevation of liver enzymes, pyrexia, and hypoglycemia[6]

Nursing Implications for Cryosurgery (Cryotherapy)

❖ Preoperative teaching is a must and includes a detailed description of the procedure and potential side effects.

❖ Assessment of the patient for treatment side effects should be ongoing.

❖ Follow-up clinical examinations include CT scan, chest x-ray, serial liver function assay, and carcinoembryonic antigen (CEA) levels. The CEA levels and CT scans are used to evaluate response to treatment.

Hepatic Artery Ligation (HAL)

❖ With the hepatic artery ligation (HAL) technique, the proper hepatic artery, or branch is ligated, resulting in cell death from hypoxia. This is only a temporary procedure, because collateral blood vessels usually form within less than a week.

❖ HAL is not routinely recommended as is has not demonstrated an impact on survival.[18]

Selective Internal Radiation Therapy (SIRT)

❖ Though this technique has been investigated in other parts of the world for many years, the FDA approved it in the U.S. in March 2002.

❖ This new technique selectively delivers high doses of radiation therapy to liver tumors.

  ❖ Small biocompatible microspheres that contain yttrium-90 and emit beta radiation are injected into the hepatic artery. The microspheres are trapped in the small blood vessels of the liver lesions where they emit their radiation.[19]

❖ Like the other targeted approaches, patients must have only liver metastatis. They cannot have any extrahepatic disease.

❖ Complications:[19]

  ❖ Fever is very common, may last for a few days to a week, and is often nocturnal.
  ❖ Abdominal pain may also be significant immediately after the procedure and may require narcotic analgesics. The pain often resolves within an hour, but may continue for several days.
  ❖ Nausea may last for several weeks and may require antiemetic therapy.
  ❖ Peptic ulceration
  ❖ Pneumonitis
  ❖ Radiation hepatitis may appear many weeks after the procedure.
  ❖ Abnormalities in liver enzymes
  ❖ An yttrium-90 SPECT scan can monitor the location of the microspheres.
  ❖ Patients can often go home the day after the procedure and resume their normal activities.

❖ Clinical research has demonstrated the benefit of this therapy:

  ❖ A phase III trial showed that the combination of the SIRT plus HAI was more effective in increasing tumor response and progression free survival as compared with HAI alone.[20]

  ❖ A phase II study reported that the addition of SIRT to a 5-FU based systemic chemotherapy regimen greatly increased both response rate and time to tumor progression as compared with the same chemotherapy alone.[21]

On the Horizon

❖ New therapies that are being investigated in primary hepatoma may eventually prove advantageous in metastatic CRC tumors. These include:

  ❖ Tumor vaccines
  ❖ Antiangiogenesis factors
  ❖ Gene therapy

Regional Approaches to Care: Nursing Implications

❖ Emotional support, symptom management, referrals for nutrition, social work, and care management are often nursing initiatives.

❖ Patient education focusing on the procedure and any preprocedure tests should be done as soon as possible. Education approaches should take into consideration the patient's learning style and coping methods as well as family/support system dynamics.

❖ Nurses may be involved in the actual delivery of treatment, as with HAI, or they may be involved in pre- and postoperative care.

References

1. Ellis L, Chase J, Patt Y, *et al.* "Hepatic Arterial Infusion Chemotherapy for Colorectal Cancer Metastasis to the Liver." In Curley S, ed. *Liver Cancer.* New York: Springer, 1998: 150–172.

2. Rychcik J. "Liver Cancer: Primary and Metastatic Disease." In Yarbro CH, Goodman M, Frogg M, *et al.*, eds. *Cancer Nursing: Principles and Practice,* 5th ed. Boston, MA: Jones and Bartlett, 2000: 1269–1297.

3. Chul HC, Radinsky R. "Biology of Colorectal Cancer Liver Metastasis." In Curley S, ed. *Liver Cancer.* New York: Springer, 1998: 212–229.

4. Wagner J, Adson M, Van Heerdon J, *et al.* "The Natural History of Hepatic Metastasis from Colorectal Cancer: A Comparison with Resective Treatment." *Ann Surg.* 1984; 199(5): 502–508.

5. Goslin R, Steele G, Zamcheck N, *et al.* "Factors Influencing Survival in Patients with Hepatic Metastasis from Adenocarcinoma of the Colon or Rectum." *Dis Colon Rectum.* 1982; 25: 749.

6. Saddler DA, and Lassere Y. "Management of Hepatic Disease." In Berg DT, ed. *Contemporary Issues in Colorectal Cancer: A Nursing Perspective.* Boston, MA: Jones and Bartlett Publishers, 2001: 203–221.

7. DeMatteo RP, Minnard EA, Kemeny N, Downey R, Burt M, Fong Y, and Blumgart LH. "Outcome after Resection of Both Liver and Lung Metastases in Patients with Colorectal Cancer." May 1999. Available at http://www.asco.org/prof/me/html/99abstracts/gic/m-958.htm. Accessed July 10, 2002.

8. Shumate C. "Hepatic Resection for Colorectal Cancer Metastases." In Curley S, ed. *Liver Cancer*. New York: Springer, 1998: 136–149.

9. Cady B, Stone M, McDermott W, et al. "Technical and Biologic Factors in Disease Free Survival after Resection for Colorectal Cancer Metastasis." *Arch Surg.* 1992; 127: 561.

10. Tuttle T. "Hepatectomy for Non-colorectal Liver Metastases." In Curley S, ed. *Liver Cancer*. New York: Springer, 1998: 201–211.

11. Reuters News. "Second Resection for Colorectal Liver Metastases Can Be Safe and Effective." June 28, 2002. Available at http://www.cancersourcern.com/news/ detail.cfm?DiseaseID=3&ContentID=25348. Accessed July 10, 2002.

12. Coia L, Ellenhorn J, and Auyoub JP. "Colorectal and Anal Cancers." In Pazdur R, Coi L, Haskins W, *et al. Cancer Management: A Multidisciplinary Approach.* Melville, NY: PRR, 2000: 273–299.

13. Kemeny N, Huang Y, Cohen AM, Shi W, Conti JA, Brennan MF, Bertino JR, Turnbull AD, Sullivan D, Stockman J, Blumgart LH, and Fong Y. "Hepatic Arterial Infusion of Chemotherapy After Resection of Hepatic Metastases from Colorectal Cancer." *New England Journal of Medicine.* 1999; 341 (27): 2039–2048.

14. Kemeny MM, Adak S, Lipsitz S, Gray B, MacDonald J, and Benson AB. "Results of the Intergroup Prospective Randomized Study of Surgery Alone Versus Continuous Hepatic Artery Infusion of FUDR and Continuous Systemic Infusion of 5-FU After Hepatic Resection for Colorectal Liver Metastasis." *Proceedings of American Society of Clinical Oncology.* 1999; 18, 264a [abstract 1012].

15. Campbell KA, Burns RC, Setzmann JV, *et al.* "Regional Chemotherapy Devices: Effect of Experience and Anatomy on Complications." *J Clin Oncol.* 1993; 11: 822–826.

16. Lencioni R, Cioni D, Goletti O, and Bartolozzi C. "Radiofrequency Thermal Ablation of Liver Tumors: State-of-the-Art." *Cancer Journal.* 2000; 6 (Suppl4): S304–S315.

17. Morris DL, King J, Zhao J, Glenn D, Clark W, and Clingan P. "Percutaneous Imaging-Guided Radio Frequency Ablation of Metastatic Colorectal Cancer in Lung." May 2002. Available at http://www.asco.org/cgi-bin/prof/abst.pl?absno=2216&div=0020&year=02abstracts. Accessed on July 8, 2002.

18. SIRteX Medical Limited. "Target Radiotherapy with SIR-spheres." Available at http://www.sirtex.com/?p=44. Accessed July 8, 2002.

19. Wagman LD, Hoff PM, Robertson J, *et al.* "Liver, Gallbladder, and Biliary Tract Cancers." In Pazdur R, Coia L, Haskins W, *et al.*, eds. *Cancer Management: A Multidisciplinary Approach.* Melville, NY: PRR, 2000: 255–271.

20. Gray B, Van Hazel G, Hope M, Burton M, Moroz P, Anderson J, and Gebski V. "Randomized Trial of SIR-Spheres Plus Chemotherapy vs. Chemotherapy Alone for Treating Patients with Liver Metastases from Primary Large Bowel Cancer." *Annals of Oncology.* 2001; 12 (12): 1711–1720.

21. Gray B, van Hazel G, Anderson J, Price D, Moroz P, Bower G, Blackwell A, and Gebski V. "Randomized Phase II Trial of SIR-Spheres Plus Fluorouracil/Leucovorin Chemotherapy Versus Fluorouracil/Leucovorin Chemotherapy Alone on Advanced Colorectal Hepatic Metastases." May 2002.

Available at http://www.asco.org/cgi-bin/prof/abst.pl ?absno=599&div=0027&year=02abstracts. Accessed on July 8, 2002.

11

Standard and Novel Systemic Treatment Options

Introduction

Approximately 25% of individuals initially diagnosed with colorectal cancer (CRC) present with metastatic disease. Unfortunately even after the best adjuvant therapy, another 50% ultimately recur, often within 2 years, with cancer in regional and/or distant sites.[1] The National Comprehensive Cancer Network (NCCN) has guidelines for treating patients with metastatic CRC. These guidelines serve as the basis for the recommendations outlined in this section.

Therapeutic Options for Metastatic Disease

❖ Carcinomas of the colon and rectum are treated differently in the adjuvant setting. In the metastatic setting, the treatment strategies are often the same.

* The treatment plan is either surgery with or without regional chemotherapy for isolated sites of metastasis or systemic chemotherapy.
* Four chemotherapy drugs are approved by the Food and Drug Administration for the systemic treatment of metastatic colorectal cancer: 5-fluorouracil (5-FU), irinotecan (CPT-11), capecitabine, and oxaliplatin. Leucovorin, frequently given in conjunction with 5-FU, is not approved by the FDA for metastatic CRC.

❖ The treatment "pathway" for patients with metastatic colorectal can appear complicated because there are many factors to consider:

* Has the primary tumor been previously resected?
* Has the patient had prior adjuvant therapy? When did they progress—within 6 months or greater than 6 months after completing adjuvant therapy?
* What is their performance status: 0–2 or ≥3? (See Appendix B)
* How many metastatic lesions are there? Are they in one organ or more than one? Are the metastases discrete lesions and therefore amendable to resection?
* Has the patient received chemotherapy for metastatic disease? If so, what did they receive, when did they receive and complete it, and how did they respond to it (both efficacy and tolerance)?
* Is the tumor progressing rapidly or growing slowly?

❖ What are the patient's wishes for treatment (one of the most important factors)?

Treatment Options for Patients Newly Diagnosed with Metastatic CRC

❖ Liver only metastases without a previous colectomy[2]

  ❖ If there are 1 to 4 discrete resectable lesions, surgery is recommended. The patient should have a colon and liver resection followed by either regional and/or systemic chemotherapy, or observation only. Regional chemotherapy would include hepatic artery infusion. Systemic chemotherapy options are noted in Table 11-1.[2]

  ❖ If the liver lesions are not amenable to surgery, NCCN recommends a palliative colon resection, especially if there is a risk of obstruction. Ablative therapy to the liver lesions may be considered. Systemic chemotherapy, noted in Table 11-1, or observation only are options.

❖ For patients with lung or abdominal metastases without a previous colectomy[2]

  ❖ If there are discrete nodules, surgery is recommended. The patient should consider a resection of the colon and the isolated metastases followed by either observation alone or systemic chemotherapy. Systemic chemotherapy could include 5-FU (infusional or bolus) and LV, with or without irinotecan, or continuous infusion 5-FU alone.[2]

TABLE 11-1
NCCN Metastatic Colorectal Cancer Practice Guidelines:
Chemotherapy Options

Regional Therapy
Hepatic artery infusion therapy ± 5-FU/leucovorin
Systemic Therapy
First-line therapy options
Irinotecan, leucovorin, bolus 5-FU
Irinotecan, leucovorin, infusional 5-FU
5-FU plus leucovorin
Continuous infusion 5-FU
Capecitabine
Second-line therapy options
Irinotecan alone
Oxaliplatin, infusional 5-FU, leucovorin[14]
Continuous infusion 5-FU
Capecitabine

- ❖ If there are multiple nodules, which are not amenable to surgery, a palliative colon resection should be considered. Systemic chemotherapy options are noted in Table 11-1.[2]

- ❖ For patients who have previously undergone a colectomy and now present with local recurrence (isolated resectable lesion[s])[2]
  - ❖ A PET scan to determine if there are any additional sites of metastatic disease is recommended.[2] If there are no additional lesions, a

resection of the metastasis is recommended followed by adjuvant systemic therapy if not given previously.[2]

❖ For patients who have had a colectomy and now have unresectable or multiple metastatic lesions there are several options depending on the individual patient:[2]

   ❖ If the patient has not had chemotherapy or if they recurred more than 6 months after adjuvant therapy and are functioning well (performance status 0–2), treatment with a clinical trial, a first-line regimen, best supportive care, or observation alone are appropriate options.[2] Systemic chemotherapy options are noted in Table 11-1. Hepatic artery infusion with or without systemic 5-FU may also be considered.[2]

    1. At the time of progression or recurrence, the patient could receive therapy on a clinical trial or a second-line treatment regimen, options noted in Table 11-1. Those who did not get treated in the first-line setting (chose best supportive care or observation) could initiate chemotherapy as appropriate.[2]

   ❖ If the patient has progressed on a first-line therapy for metastatic disease or if they recurred within 6 months after adjuvant therapy and have a performance status of 0–2, treatment with a clinical trial or on a second-line regimen is recommended, noted in Table 11-1.[2]

❖ If the patient has not received prior chemotherapy but is functioning poorly (performance status ≥3), the NCCN recommends best supportive care.[2]

Information of the Approaches to Care

❖ 5-FU plus LV
  ❖ 5-FU is a thymidine synthetase inhibitor. LV is a vitamin (folinic acid).
  ❖ 5-FU and LV became the standard chemotherapy regimen for untreated CRC in 1992 when it was shown to be superior to 5-FU alone.[3]
  ❖ 5-FU and LV may be given in either a bolus or continuous intravenous infusion schedule. Bolus schedules are common in the U.S. and research was built on this platform. In Europe, the continuous intravenous infusion method is used and is the basis for their research.
  ❖ The efficacy of the two bolus regimens (Mayo and Roswell Park) is equivalent. The various infusional regimens are considered comparable in terms of efficacy. When bolus schedules are compared with continuous infusion schedules, the bolus schedules are felt to be more toxic, while the continuous infusion schedules are considered more efficacious. A summarization of this is noted in Table 11-2.[4,5]
  ❖ Common dosing: the common regimens are illustrated in Table 11-3 (note dosing varies widely).
  ❖ The common toxicities (depend on the schedule): stomatitis, bone marrow suppression, diarrhea, and ocular changes (e.g., blurred

TABLE 11-2
Efficacy of Common 5 cm and LV Regimens

	Mayo Regimen (bolus)	Roswell Park Regimen (bolus)	de Gramont Regimen (infusional)	Meta-analysis Bolus	Meta-analysis Infusional
Response Rate (RR)	35%	31%	32.6%	14%	22%
Overall survival (OS)	9.3 mos.	10.7 mos.	14.1 mo.	11.3 mos.	12.1 mos.

TABLE 11-3
Common Metastatic Chemotherapy Regimens

Drug/Combination	Dose and Schedule
Irinotecan, leucovorin, and bolus 5-FU (bolus IFL)	
[first line therapy]	
Irinotecan	125 mg/m^2 IV over 90 minutes
Leucovorin	20 mg/m^2 IV bolus
5-FU	500 mg/m^2 IV push
	Repeated weekly × 4 weeks every 6 weeks
	Though not the FDA-approved dose, irinotecan and 5-FU starting doses may be reduced to 100 mg/m^2 and 400 mg/m^2 respectively.
Irinotecan, leucovorin, and infusional 5-FU (infusional IFL)	
[first line therapy]	
Irinotecan	180 mg/m^2 IV over 90 minutes day 1 every 2 weeks
Leucovorin	200 mg/m^2 IV over 2 hours, followed by
5-FU	400 mg/m^2 IV push, then 600 mg/m^2 CI over 22 hours
	Leucovorin and 5-FU are repeated days 1 and 2
	Cycle repeats every 2 weeks

TABLE 11-3
Common Metastatic Chemotherapy Regimens (continued)

Drug/Combination	Dose and Schedule
5-fluorouracil (5-FU) plus low-dose leucovorin (Mayo [bolus])	
Leucovorin	20 mg/m^2 IV bolus just prior to 5-FU for 5 consecutive days
5-FU	425 mg/m^2 IV push for 5 consecutive days
	Repeated every 28 days
5-fluorouracil (5-FU) plus high-dose leucovorin (Roswell Park [bolus])	
Leucovorin	500 mg/m^2 IV over 2 hours
5-FU	500–700 mg/m^2 IV push given 1 hour after start of leucovorin
	Repeated weekly for 6 weeks followed by 2 weeks rest
Infusional 5-FU plus leucovorin (de Gramont)	
Leucovorin	200 mg/m^2 IV over 2 hours, followed by
5-FU	400 mg/m^2 IV push, then 600 mg/m^2 CI over 22 hours
	Repeated days 1 and 2 every 2 weeks

(continued)

TABLE 11-3
Common Metastatic Chemotherapy Regimens (continued)

Drug/Combination	Dose and Schedule
Infusional 5-FU (Lockich)	
5-FU	300 mg/m² CI every day
Infusional high-dose 5-FU plus leucovorin (AIO)	
Leucovorin	500 mg/m² IV over 2 hours
5-FU	2,600 mg/m² IV over 24 hours
	Repeat weekly × 6 weeks every 8 weeks
Capecitabine	1250mg/m² PO BID day 1–14 every 3 weeks
	Though not FDA approved, the dose may also start at 1000mg/m².
Irinotecan (single agent; second line therapy)	125 mg/m² IV over 90 minutes weekly for 4 weeks, then 2 weeks rest; *or*
	350 mg/m² IV over 90 minutes once every 3 weeks

(continued)

TABLE 11-3
Common Metastatic Chemotherapy Regimens (continued)

Drug/Combination	Dose and Schedule
Oxaliplatin, leucovorin, and infusional 5-FU (FOLFOX 4) (second line therapy)	
Oxaliplatin	85 mg/m^2 IV over 2–6 hours on day 1
Leucovorin	200 mg/m^2 IV over 2 hours on days 1 and 2
5-FU	400 mg/m^2 IV push, then 600 mg/m2 IV over 22 hours on days 1 and 2
	Repeated every 2 weeks
Irinotecan, leucovorin, and infusional 5-FU (FOLFIRI) [Investigational]	
Irinotecan	180 mg/m^2 IV over 90 minutes on day 1
Leucovorin	200 mg/m^2 IV over 2 hours on day 1
5-FU	400 mg/m^2 IV push on day 1, then 2.4 to 3 g/m^2 IV over 46 hours
	Repeated every 2 weeks

(continued)

TABLE 11-3
Common Metastatic Chemotherapy Regimens (continued)

Drug/Combination	Dose and Schedule
Oxaliplatin, leucovorin, and infusional 5-FU [FOLFOX [modified]] [Investigational]	
Oxaliplatin	100 mg/m^2 IV over 2–6 hours on day 1
Leucovorin	200 mg/m^2 IV over 2 hours on day 1
5-FU	400 mg/m^2 IV push on day 1, then 2.4 to 3 g/m^2 IV over 46 hours
	Repeated every 2 weeks

vision). In addition, nausea, vomiting, hair loss, changes in nails, skin reactions (e.g., sun sensitivity, hand and foot syndrome), cerebellar alterations, and increased tearing have been reported but are infrequent. *Note:* stomatitis and neutropenia are more common with the Mayo regimen; diarrhea is more common with the Roswell Park regimen; and hand-foot syndrome is associated with continuous infusion regimens.[4,5]

- ❖ Special considerations: doses should be reduced in patients with hepatic, renal, or bone marrow abnormalities. A central venous access device and ambulatory pump are required to administer continuous infusion 5-FU.

❖ Irinotecan

- ❖ Irinotecan is a topoisomerase I inhibitor.
- ❖ Irinotecan, as a single agent, was approved as a second-line therapy in 1998.

  1. It demonstrated significant improvement in response rate and progression-free survival as compared to best supportive care or infusional 5-FU.[6,7]

- ❖ In 2000, irinotecan in combination with 5-FU and LV was approved by the FDA as a first line treatment for metastatic CRC.

  1. In two phase III clinical trials, one using bolus 5-FU, LV, and irinotecan (bolus IFL); the other using continuous infusion 5-FU, LV and irinotecan (infusional IFL), both

TABLE 11–4
Efficacy of Two Irinotecan, 5 FU plus LV Regimens

	Bolus IFL vs Mayo		Infusional IFL vs Infusional 5-FU/LV	
RR	39%	21%	35%	22%
PFS	7.0 mos.	4.3 mos.	6.7 mos.	4.4 mos.
OS	14.8 mos.	12.6 mos.	17.4 mos.	14.1 mos.

demonstrated significant improvement in response rate (RR), progression-free survival (PFS), and overall survival (OS).[8,9] The results are shown in Table 11-4.

❖ Usual dose range: the dose and schedule varies whether it is used first or second line. See common regimens in Table 11-3.

❖ Common toxicities: diarrhea, bone marrow suppression, nausea, vomiting, hair loss, and cholinergic reaction (e.g., increased sweating, tearing, abdominal cramping). Infrequently mouth sores and mild rashes have been reported.[8,9,10]

❖ Special considerations: The manufacturer recommends increased monitoring of patients for toxicity and dose modifications based on their tolerance. Toxicity may be more severe in patients who are functioning poorly (performance status ≥2).[10] Other considerations include changing the schedule of the bolus IFL regimen to days 1 and 8 every 3 weeks; administer IFL by the infusional schedule which is FDA approved, or decrease the starting doses of the irinotecan and 5-FU in the bolus schedule.[2]

❖ Capecitabine

  ❖ Capecitabine is an inhibitor of thymidylate synthetase. The molecule is ultimately converted to 5-FU through activation by thymidine phosphorylase (TP), an enzyme that is overexpressed in tumor cells.

  ❖ In 2001, capecitabine was approved by the FDA for patients with metastatic CRC when 5-FU alone therapy is preferred. The capecitabine studies were ongoing when the FDA approved the IFL combination; therefore, the FDA noted that the combination therapy improved survival over 5-FU and LV (Mayo) and capecitabine did not. Moreover, the FDA also stated that substitution of capecitabine for the 5-FU in an IFL regimen still needs to be proven in clinical trials and cannot be recommended at this time.[12]

  ❖ Phase III clinical trial results are noted in Table 11-5 (abbreviations: response rate [RR], time to

TABLE 11-5
Efficacy in Phase III Trial Comparing Capecitabine to 5-FU and LV (Mayo)

	Capecitabine	Mayo Regimen
RR	25.8%	11.6%
TTP	4.3 mos.	4.7 mos.
OS	12.5 mos.	13.3 mos.

tumor progression [TTP], and overall survival [OS]).[11,12]

❖ Usual dose range is 1000–1250 mg/m² PO BID days 1–14 every 3 weeks.

❖ Common toxicities: hand and foot syndrome, hyperbilirubinema, diarrhea, nausea, vomiting, stomatitis, abdominal pain, constipation, anorexia, and fatigue. Bone marrow suppression, alopecia, increased tearing, headaches, and dizziness can occur but are infrequent.[12]

❖ Special considerations: Patient compliance is a concern, both in taking this oral medication and in stopping it in the face of moderate toxicity. Patients with severe renal impairment should not take capecitabine. Patients with elevated bilirubin levels should have doses of capecitabine decreased. Also folic acid, including leucovorin, should not be taken concomitantly with capecitabine. Patients taking medications that affect blood clotting should be monitored closely for abnormalities in coagulation studies. Toxicity may be severe in the older patient.[12]

❖ Platinum compound: oxaliplatin

❖ Oxaliplatin inhibits DNA replication and transcription by forming intrastrand DNA crosslinks, a mechanism similar to other platinum agents–cisplatin and carboplatin.[13]

- ❖ In August 2002, the FDA approved the combination of oxaliplatin, 5-FU and LV in the treatment of patients whose CRC recurred or progressed during or within 6 months following standard first-line treatment with irinotecan, 5FU, plus LV.[14]

    1. In a multi-center phase III trial, oxaliplatin, 5-FU, and LV was shown to significantly shrink CRC tumors as compared to 5-FU and LV or oxaliplatin alone (objective response rate 9%, 0%, and 1% respectively).[14]

    2. This trial also demonstrated a significant delay in the time it took the tumors to regrow with the combination as compared with 5-FU and LV or oxaliplatin alone (time to tumor progression 4.6 months, 2.7 months, and 1.6 months respectively).[14]

    3. At the time of the FDA approval, no data was available on the effect of the combination on overall survival.[14]

    4. The FDA approval was an accelerated approval; therefore, more data is pending.[14]

- ❖ Because oxaliplatin is approved in Europe, as the first- and second-line treatment of CRC, there is a large body of evidence about its activity. The majority of research studies show a significant benefit in tumor response, but in none did this translate into statistically better survival.[15] In patients who have not received prior chemotherapy, the response is approximately 27% for oxaliplatin alone and

57% when combined with 5-FU. For those previously treated, the response rates are lower generally, 10% for oxaliplatin alone and 45% for oxaliplatin plus 5-FU.[15]

❖ A summarization of three randomized trials is noted in Table 11-6 (abbreviations: response rate [RR], progression free survival [PFS], overall survival [OS], infusional 5-FU, LV, oxaliplatin [FOLFOX-4], infusional 5-FU and LV [de Gramont], modified infusional 5-FU, LV, irinotecan[FOLFIRI], modified infusional 5-FU, LV, oxaliplatin [FOLFOX], irinotecan, leucovorin, bolus 5-FU [bolus IFL]).[16,17,18]

❖ There are controversies about the U.S. trial comparing bolus IFL to FOLFOX4, shown in Table 11-6, many of which are interrelated.[18,19]

1. Despite the difference in response rate and survival, the time to treatment failure was equal in both treatments (5.5 months and 5.8 months, respectively).

2. More patients were removed from therapy due to toxicity on the oxaliplatin containing arm (55% FOLFOX 4 versus 30% bolus IFL).

3. This translated into more patients receiving an FDA approved/effective second-line therapy on the FOLFOX 4 arm as compared with bolus IFL (52% on FOLFOX 4 received irinotecan second line whereas only 17% of those on bolus IFL received oxaliplatin second line), as oxaliplatin was still investigational during this study.

TABLE 11-6

Oxaliplatin, 5FU, and LV as First-Line Treatment of Matastatic CRC: Summary of Three Phase III Trials

	FOLFOX 4	de Gramont	FOLFIRI	FOLFOX	Bolus IFL	FOLFOX 4
RR	50.7% *	22.3%	56%	54%	29%	38%*
PFS	9.0 mos.*	6.2 mos.	14.4 mos.	11.5 mos.	6.9 mos.	8.8 mos.*
OS	16.2 mos.	14.7 mos.	20.4 mos.	21.5 mos.	14.1 mos.	18.6 mos.*

*Difference is statistically significant.

4. The definition of time to tumor progression was not standard in this study and permitted change of therapy for reasons other than progression while scoring the duration of response to the initial treatment. (Patients were not censored when they discontinued therapy for toxicity and then started a second-line therapy; instead the remission was counted through the additional therapy but attributed to the first-line treatment.)

❖ Usual dose:

1. FDA approved regimen: Oxaliplatin plus infusional 5-FU and LV. See Table 11-3 for details.[14]
2. Single agent, either: 85 mg/m^2 IV every 2 weeks or 130 mg/m^2 IV every 3 weeks. It is administered intravenously over 2 to 6 hours. Variations may be prescribed in the clinical trial.[13]

❖ Common toxicities: cold-induced peripheral sensory neuropathy (numbness and tingling in hands and feet), acute laryngopharyngeal dysesthesia, nausea, vomiting, diarrhea, abdominal cramping, neutropenia, thrombocytopenia, and fatigue. Infrequently reported are allergic reactions, stomatitis, and pulmonary fibrosis.[14]

Emerging Directions in the Treatment of Metastatic CRC

❖ Vascular endothelial growth factor inhibitors: bevacizumab

  ❖ Bevacizumab (rhuMAb-VEGF, Avastin) is an investigational recombinant humanized monoclonal antibody that binds to vascular endothelial growth factor (VEGF) receptors. This binding interferes with signals into the cell which normally tells the endothelial cell to divide and make new blood vessels; when inhibited, the signals are not received and new blood vessels are not made.

  ❖ An early phase II trial looking at two doses of bevacizumab plus 5-FU and LV and 5-FU plus LV alone showed a benefit for the addition of bevacizumab. Two phase III clinical trials are underway: one comparing bolus IFL with or without bevacizumab, the other comparing 5-FU plus LV with or without bevacizumab.[20]

  ❖ Usual dose: 5–10 mg/kg IV every 2 weeks or as prescribed in the clinical trial.[20]

  ❖ Common toxicities: hypersensitivity reactions, acute hypertension, thrombosis, bleeding, and headache[21]

❖ Epideral growth factor receptor inhibitors: cetuximab (IMC-C225) and iressa

  ❖ The epideral growth factor receptor (EGFR) promotes cell growth and differentiation through the signaling pathway to tyrosine kinase within the cell. EGFR inhibitors bind to receptors on the cell membrane, inhibiting signals to the inside of the cell, thereby blocking cell growth. EGFR is overexpressed in many tumor types, including CRC where it has been found in approximately 25–77% of CRC tumors.[21] There are two EGFR inhibitors being investigated in CRC: IMC-C225 and iressa.

❖ Cetuximab (IMC-C225; C225)

1. There have been two clinical trials reported which demonstrate the activity of C225 in metastatic CRC. Both phase II trials treated patients whose disease had progressed on irinotecan therapy with either C225 alone or C225 added to irinotecan. As a single agent, C225 produced a response rate of 10.5%.[22] In combination with irinotecan, the response rate was 22.5%.[22] A phase III trial in first-line metastatic CRC is planned.

2. Usual dose: C225 test dose of 20 mg/10mL IV over 10 minutes. If after a 30-minute observation period there are no allergic reactions, then the loading dose is administered. Loading dose 400mg/m^2 over 120 minutes, followed by weekly doses of 250 mg/m^2 over 60 minutes.[22] Variations may be prescribed in the clinical trial.

3. Common toxicities: acne-like rash and allergic reaction are the clinically significant side effects. Additional toxicities include nausea, vomiting, diarrhea, fatigue, fever, neutrope-

nia, and increased serum alanine amino-transferase (ALT or SGPT).[13]

❖ Iressa (ZD1839)

1. There is both laboratory and early clinical evidence that iressa has activity in metastatic CRC. In one early clinical study, iressa was given in combination with 5-FU and LV. The investigators noted activity without an increase in toxicity.[21] The next phase of clinical trials comparing standard chemotherapy alone or with the addition of iressa are being planned.

2. Usual dose: 250–500 mg PO per day or as prescribed in the clinical trial.[20]

3. Common toxicities: nausea, vomiting, bone pain, fatigue, diarrhea, and an acne-like rash[21]

❖ Antiangiogenesis agent: thalidomide

  ❖ Thalidomide is an investigational agent. Although its exact mechanism of action is unclear, it is believed to be an antiangiogenesis agent.[23]

  ❖ Early clinical trials have suggested an improvement in toxicity, specifically diarrhea, when thalidomide was combined with irinotecan.[13,23,24] One of those trials was recently updated, and the authors reported a 30% response rate in 5-FU refractory patients when treated with irinotecan and thalidomide. Less grade 3/4 toxicity (severe hematological [18%], late onset diarrhea [11%], nausea and vomiting [14%]) was also noted. Additional clinical trials are underway to further determine its dose and role in CRC.[24]

- ❖ Usual dose: 200–400 mg/day at bedtime or as prescribed in the clinical trial.[24]
- ❖ Common toxicities: teratogenicity, sedation, constipation, peripheral neuropathy, deep vein thrombosis, pulmonary embolus, and skin rash[23]

❖ Cyclooxygenase-2 (COX-2) inhibitors: celecoxib and rofecoxib

- ❖ Laboratory research has demonstrated that COX-2 plays a role in carcinogenesis possibly by the promotion of angiogenesis, induction of cellular proliferation, and the inhibition of apoptosis. Laboratory research has also demonstrated that the inhibition of COX-2, especially by specific inhibitors, can reverse these effects leading to a decrease in cellular growth.[24] COX-2 is overexpressed in all major cancers, including CRC; therefore, there is a target for the therapy. Because there are no overlapping toxicities between the COX-2 inhibitors and current chemotherapy agents, many clinical trials are being developed combining these two treatment methods.[25]
- ❖ Rofecoxib

  1. One recent clinical trial added rofecoxib to the Mayo regimen of 5-FU and LV. Two of the first three patients suffered gastrointestinal bleeding (GI) necessitating a decrease in the rofecoxib dosage. Even after the dose

decrease, there was additional GI bleeding. The authors also did not see any responses with this therapy and therefore concluded that rofecoxib does not improve upon chemotherapy alone but adds to toxicity.[26]

2. Usual dose: 25–50 mg/day PO[26]
3. Common toxicities (rofecoxib alone): edema, hypertension, heart failure, stomach ulcers, GI bleeding, diarrhea, nausea, and heartburn[27]

❖ Celecoxib

1. Three recent clinical trials relating specifically to CRC were reported. Two trials combined celecoxib to the standard chemotherapy of bolus IFL.[28,29] The third trial was a retrospective analysis of patients on capecitabine who either also took celecoxib for pain or not.[30] Though the results are preliminary on all three trials, celecoxib use may lead to a decrease in toxicity from standard chemotherapy (two trials reported a decrease in neutropenia, the third trial reported a significant decrease in capecitabine-induced hand foot syndrome), leading to an enhanced efficacy or improved quality of life. Efficacy of the regimens was also reported in all three trials though the number of patients participating was small. Further research is needed to clarify the role of celecoxib in the treatment of CRC.

2. Usual dose: 400 mg PO BID

3. Common toxicities (celecoxib alone): indigestion, diarrhea, and abdominal pain. In rare cases, serious stomach problems, such as bleeding, can occur without warning.[31]

Future Directions

❖ The treatment of metastatic CRC is an active field. Future strategies are looking at combining the FDA-approved agents with each other, with the new cytotoxic agents, and with the molecularly targeted agents. The result is many different treatment options for patients. For example, one clinical trial under development is proposing to compare infusional 5-FU, LV, plus irinotecan to infusional 5-FU, LV, plus oxaliplatin. Patients in both arms would then also be randomized to receive C225 or placebo. Other trials are looking at the other molecularly targeted agents instead, e.g., iressa, celecoxib.

❖ In addition, specific agents may be chosen for an individual patient based on their tumor's (pharmacogenomics) characteristics. "Tailored" therapy may become a reality.

References

1. Guillem JG, Paty PB, and Cohen AM. "Surgical Treatment of Colorectal Cancer." *CA: Cancer J Clin.* 1997; 47(2):113–128.

2. National Comprehensive Cancer Network (NCCN). "Colon and Rectal Cancer Treatment Guidelines." *The*

Complete Library of Practice Guidelines in Oncology, 2nd ed. Version 2001. Rockledge, PA: NCCN, 2001.

3. Fuchs CS, and Mayer RJ. "Colorectal Cancer Chemotherapy." In Rustgi AK, ed. *Gastrointestinal Cancers: Biology, Diagnosis, and Therapy*. Boston, MA: Lippincott Williams & Wilkins, 1995: 423–442.

4. Meta-analysis Group in Cancer. "Efficacy of Intravenous Continuous Infusion of Fluorouracil Compared with Bolus Administration in Advanced Colorectal Cancer." *Journal of Clinical Oncology*. 1998; 16: 301–308.

5. Buroker TR, O'Connell MJ, Wieand HS, Krook JE, Gerstner JB, Mailliard JA, Schaefer PL, Levitt R, Kardinal CG, and Gesme DH. "Randomized Comparison of Two Schedules of Fluorouracil and Leucovorin in the Treatment of Advanced Colorectal Cancer." *Journal of Clinical Oncology*. 1994; 12: 14–20.

6. Cunningham D, Pyrhonen S, James RD, *et al.* "Randomized Trial of Irinotecan Plus Supportive Care Versus Supportive Care Alone After Fluorouracil Failure for Patients with Metastatic Colorectal Cancer." *Lancet*. 1998; 352 (9138): 1413–1418.

7. Rougier P, Van Cutsem E, Bajetta E, *et al.* "Randomized Trial of Irinotecan Versus Fluorouracil by Continuous Infusion After Fluorouracil Failure in Patients with Metastatic Colorectal Cancer." *Lancet*. 1998; 352(9138): 1407–1412.

8. Saltz LB, Cox JV, Blanke C, *et al.*, for the Irinotecan Study Group. "Irinotecan Plus Fluorouracil and Leucovorin for Metastatic Colorectal Cancer." *New England Journal of Medicine*. 2000; 343(13): 905–914.

9. Douillard JY, Cunningham D, Roth AD, *et al.* "Irinotecan Combined with Fluorouracil Compared with Fluorouracil Alone as First-Line Treatment for

Metastatic Colorectal Cancer: A Multicentre Randomised Trial." *Lancet*. 2000: 355: 1041–1047.

10. Pharmacia Oncology. Camptosar (irinotecan hydrochloride) [package insert]. Peapack, NJ: Pharmacia Oncology, 2002.

11. Cassidy J, Twelves C, Van Cutsem E, Hoff P, Bajetta E, Boyer M, Bugat R, Burger U, Garin A, Graeven U, McKendrick J, Maroun J, Marshall J, Osterwalder B, Perez-Manga G, Rosso R, Rougier P, and Schilsky RL. "First-line Oral Capecitabine Therapy in Metastatic Colorectal Cancer: A Favorable Safety Profile Compared with Intravenous 5-Fluorouracil/Leucovorin." *Annals of Oncology*. 2002; 13: 566–575.

12. Roche Laboratories, Inc. Xeloda (capecitabine) tablets [package insert]. Nutley, NJ: Roche Laboratories, Inc. Available at www.xeloda.com/XELODA-PI.html. Accessed June 28, 2002.

13. Berg DT, and Lilienfeld C. "Therapeutic Options for Treating Advanced Colorectal Cancer." *Clinical Journal of Oncology Nursing*. 2000; 4(5): 209–216.

14. FDA. Eloxatin™ (oxaliplatin for injection). Available at http://www.fda.gov/cder/drug/infopage/eloxatin. Accessed August 15, 2002.

15. Goldberg RM. "Gastrointestinal Tract Cancers." In Casciato DA. And Lowitz BB, eds. *Manual of Clinical Oncology*, 4th ed. Philadelphia, PA: Lippincott Williams & Wilkins. 2000: 182–194.

16. De Gramont A, Figer A, Seymour M, *et al.* "Leucovorin and Fluorouracil with or Without Oxaliplatin as First-Line Treatment in Advanced Colorectal Cancer." *Journal of Clinical Oncology*. 2000; 18(16): 2938–2947.

17. Tournigand C, Louvet C, Quinaux E, *et al.* "FOLFIRI Followed by FOLFOX Versus FOLFOX Followed by FOLFIRI in Metastatic Colorectal Cancer: Final Results

of a Phase III Study." Proceedings of ASCO. 2001; 20: 124a, abstract 494.

18. Goldberg RM, Morton RF, Sargent DJ, *et al.* "N9741: Oxaliplatin or CPT-11 + 5-Fluorouracil/Leucovorin or Oxaliplatin+ CPT-11 in Advanced Colorectal Cancer: Initial Toxicity and Response Data from a GI Intergroup Study." Proceedings of ASCO. 2001; 20: 128a, abstract 511.

19. Haller DG. "Colorectal Cancer Treatment of Advanced Disease and Adjuvant Therapy." May 20, 2002. Available at http://virtualmeeting.asco.org/vm2002/gastro.cfm. Accessed June 30, 2002.

20. "National Cancer Institute Cancer Clinical Trials." Available at http://cancer.gov. Accessed June 30, 2002.

21. CancersourceRN.com. "2002 Oncology Nursing Drug Database." Available at http://www.cancersourcern.com/drugdb/index.cfm. Accessed June 28, 2002.

22. Saltz L, Meropol NJ, Loehrer PJ, *et al.* "Single Agent IMC-C225 Has Activity In CPT-11-Refractory Colorectal Cancer That Expresses the Epidermal Growth Factor Receptor." Proceedings of ASCO. 2002; 20: 127a, abstract 504.

23. Nirenberg A. "Thalidomide: When Everything Old Is New Again." *Clinical Journal of Oncology Nursing.* 2001: 5(1): 15–18.

24. Govindarajan R, Maddox AM, Safar AM, *et al.* "The Efficacy of Thalidomide and Irinotecan in Metastatic Colorectal Carcinoma (Phase II Study)." *Proceedings of ASCO.* 2002; 20: 102b, abstract 2222.

25. Soslow RA, Dannenberg AJ, Rush D, *et al.* "COX-2 Is Expressed in Human Pulmonary, Colonic and Mammary Tumors." *Cancer.* 2000; 89(12): 2637–2645.

26. Becerra EP, Frenket R, and Gaynor R. "A Phase II Study of 5-Fluorouracil and Leucovorin Calcium Plus Open-Label Rofecoxib in Patients with Metastatic Colorectal Cancer." *Proceedings of ASCO.* 2002; 20: 107b, abstract 2240.

27. Food and Drug Administration. "Consumer Information: Rofecoxib." Available at http://www.fda.gov/cder/consumerinfo/druginfo/vioxx .htm. Accessed June 26, 2002.

28. Blanke CD, Benson AB, Dragovich T, *et al.* "A Phase II Trial of Celecoxib, Irinotecan, 5-Fluorouracil, and Leucovorin in Patients with Unresectable or Metastatic Colorectal Cancer." *Proceedings of ASCO.* 2002; 20: 127a, abstract 505.

29. Sweeney C, Seitz D, Ansari R., *et al.* A Phase II Trial of Irinotecan, 5-Fluorouracil, Leucovorin, Celecoxib and Glutamine as First Line Therapy for Advanced Colorectal Cancer: A Hoosier Oncology Group Study." *Proceedings of ASCO.* 2002; 20: 105b, abstract 2235.

30. Lin EH, Morris J, Chau NK, *et al.* "Celecoxib Attenuated Capecitabine Induced Hand-and-Foot Syndrome and Diarrhea and Improved Time to Tumor Progression in Metastatic Colorectal Cancer." *Proceedings of ASCO.* 2002; 20: 138b, abstract 2364.

31. Pharmacia. Celebrex (celecoxib) [package insert]. Peapack, NJ: Pharmacia, 2002. Available at http://www.celebrex.com/celebrex-facts.asp#a7. Accessed June 29, 2002.

PART V

Care of the Individual with Colorectal Cancer

12

Treatment Toxicities and Symptom Management: Considerations for Nursing Practice

Introduction

The etiology of toxicities and symptoms associated with colorectal cancer result from the disease process, treatment, and/or a combination of these two. The effective management of the toxicities and symptoms is derived from many sources, including a working knowledge of evidenced-based interventions and creativity. The goal of this section is to provide a practical approach to the management of the common treatment-related toxicities and symptoms.

Symptom Assessment

❖ A *symptom* is the individual's subjective experience of the physical and emotional disturbances related to the disease process and/or the treatment for the disease itself.

❖ Assessment of *symptom occurrence* includes the following:

- ❖ Onset of the symptom: Is the symptom new, or has it occurred before?
- ❖ Pattern of the symptom: Constant versus intermittent?
- ❖ Location: Patient's perception of the anatomic location
- ❖ Aggravating and alleviating factors: "What seems to make it worse and what seems to make it better?"
- ❖ Severity: Some symptoms can be measured, while others are more subjective. This is perhaps the most elusive component of symptom assessment. Consistently using the same scale, whether it be the National Cancer Institute's Common Toxicity Criteria or another measure is key.
- ❖ Use of complementary therapies: May be the cause of abnormal symptoms

❖ *Symptom distress:* The amount of anguish that occurs as result of a symptom.[1] "How much does the symptom bother you (use the same numerical, descriptive, or pictorial scale to elicit symptom severity)?"

Care of the Patient with Advanced Colorectal Cancer

❖ Knowledge deficit regarding disease process and treatment plan

Nursing Interventions:

- ❖ Assess the patient's understanding of the diagnosis and the treatment options.
- ❖ Ascertain the patient's and family's willingness to learn and comply with the treatment regimen.
- ❖ Educate the patient regarding the treatment's purpose, schedule, common side effects, and self-care measures to manage side effects.
- ❖ Review with the patient and family when to call for medical/nursing advice.

❖ Nausea and vomiting

Nursing Interventions:

- ❖ Assess the likelihood of nausea and vomiting based on several factors:
  1. Emetogenic potential of the treatment
  2. Individual characteristics associated with higher risk of emesis: female gender, younger age, and history of motion sickness
  3. Individual characteristics associated with lower risk, e.g., chronic alcohol intake
  4. Nfactor, interactive program to determine emetogenic potential of chemotherapy and/or radiation therapy, may be helpful. Accessible at http://www.kytril.com/nfactor/

index.asp. *Note:* 5-FU, irinotecan, and oxali-platin are considered moderately emetogenic; capecitabine has a low emetogenic potential, but risk may increase with multimodality or combination therapy.

❖ Evaluate the potential impact of comorbid conditions
❖ Identify the underlying cause of the symptom, i.e., acute, delayed, anticipatory, or refractory and initiate appropriate corrective measures
❖ Proactively administer antiemetics prior to therapy and regularly thereafter. Select a regimen based on the emetogenic potential of the therapy. See Table 12-1.
❖ Evaluate and adjust the antiemetic regimen according to patient tolerance

  1. Assess the symptom and level of distress, encouraging the patient to record frequency of emesis

❖ Incorporate nonpharmacologic interventions, such as accupressure, guided imagery, and music therapy
❖ Encourage dietary modifications

  1. Eat small, bland meals without unpleasant odors or tastes
  2. Cool, cold, or room temperature foods are often tolerated better.
  3. Clear liquids, carbonated sodas, crackers, or dry toast can be helpful.
  4. Change the diet to clear liquids if vomiting is experienced.

TABLE 12-1
Antiemetic Agents[30]

Drug	Dose and Frequency
Dexamethasone	10–20 mg IV or 4mg PO pretreatment and q 4–6 hours PRN
Prochlorperazine	5–25 mg PO q 4–6; 10–75 mg q 12h (slow release). IV 10–20 mg. IM/PR dosing also available, but not usually required.
Ondansetron	8–32 mg IV, 8–32 mg PO beginning 30 minutes before treatment. Oral dosing may be repeated BID for 1–2 days.
Granisetron	10 μg/kg IV 30 minutes before treatment; or 2 mg PO once daily or 1 mg PO twice daily (second dose given 12 hours after the first) beginning 60 minutes before treatment. Regimens given day of chemotherapy only, as continued treatment has not been found to be effective.
Dolasetron	100 mg IV or PO. IV dosing may also be calculated at 1.8 mg/kg. Administer 30 minutes before treatment.

Note: dexamethasone 10–20 mg PO or IV and/or lorazepam 1–6 mg PO may be given along with serotonin antagonist.

❖ Bone marrow suppression

Nursing Interventions:

   ❖ Monitor complete blood count (CBC) before each cycle of therapy and regularly in-between as appropriate

* Calculate absolute neutrophil count (ANC) by the following formula:
  Segmented neutrophils (%) + bands (%) x white blood cell count = ANC.
* Delay chemotherapy dose as recommended depending on the CBC/ANC results
* Modify subsequent doses of chemotherapy based on the lowest ANC during the cycle
* According to ASCO guidelines for growth factors, prophylactic use is not recommended in this patient population, but may be considered in select patients.[2]

❖ Mucositis or stomatitis

Nursing Interventions:

* Perform a baseline oral mucosal examination and reevaluate with each treatment
* Consider cryotherapy for the prevention of 5-fluorouracil-induced mucositis; ask the patient to suck on ice chips for 5 minutes before the bolus injection and for at least 25 minutes afterward. **Do not** recommend cryotherapy for patients receiving oxaliplatin.
* Teach the patient to perform an oral examination and to report change
* Instruct the patient to cleanse the mouth at least twice a day, rinsing with nonirritating, plain- or sterile-water mouth rinses three to four times during the day; Prevention is key. Simple measures are effective.

- Assess and adjust the interventions according to effectiveness
- Consider the use of sucralfate, antifungal agents, antiviral agents, and/or topical or systemic pain medications that can be added on an individual basis if symptoms worsen
- Advise the patient to stop wearing dentures if oral ulcers are present
- Encourage the patient to eat soft or liquid foods high in protein and avoid alcohol, citrus fruits, acidy juices, spicy foods, tobacco, and commercial mouthwashes
- Consider the need for delay or dose modification with the physician

- Taste changes and anorexia

Nursing Interventions:

- Assess the etiology of symptoms and develop a plan to correct the underlying cause
- Assess the patient's baseline dietary intake, concomitant medications, and any gastrointestinal symptoms or abnormalities that may impact the problem
- Monitor the patient's weight and report any weight loss or gain
- Teach the patient to cleanse his or her mouth before and after meals
- Suggest that the patient experiment with seasonings, salt, sorbitol, and sweetened candies (mints, hard candy, or cough drops) to make food more appealing and palatable[3]

* If nausea is present, administer antiemetics before mealtime
* Encourage the patient to eat foods at room temperature or cold, small, frequent meals instead of three large meals, foods high in protein and calories, limit liquids during eating, and maximize intake when feeling the best.
* Encourage the patient to establish a pleasant, unhurried environment for mealtime
* Advise the patient's family and friends against preparing and forcing the patient's favorite foods during periods of severe taste changes and/or nausea. These may be subsequently associated with the adverse symptoms.[3]
* Offer liquid food supplements if the patient is not tolerating solid foods
* Initiate pharmacologic interventions, such as corticosteroids, megestrol acetate, hydrazine sulfate, metoclopramide, and dronabinol, as ordered

❖ Constipation

Nursing Interventions:

* Assess the patient's baseline bowel habits and concomitant medications
* Identify the underlying cause of constipation and initiate interventions based on cause
* Educate the patient about pharmacologic and dietary means to prevent constipation
* Advise the patient:[4]
    1. Not to strain with bowel movements
    2. To respond immediately to the urge to defecate

3. To create privacy and plenty of time for the bowel routine

❖ Increase fiber intake, whole-grain foods, legumes, fresh foods, and raw vegetables, unless contraindicated[4]

❖ Increase fluid intake; recommend 2 to 3 quarts of liquids including juices, water, and prune juice. A hot beverage first thing in the morning may be helpful.[4]

❖ Follow a prescribed bowel regimen to prevent or manage opioid-induced constipation as per the physician's or nurse's instructions[4]

❖ Report to the physician or nurse any changes in abdomen or bowel movements lasting for 3 days

❖ Assess the abdomen for bowel sounds, fecal impaction, and possible advancement to bowel obstruction

❖ Diarrhea

Nursing Interventions:

❖ Assess the patient's baseline bowel habits, concomitant medications, past history of constipation and/or diarrhea, and the diarrheal potential of the chemotherapy regimen; continue assessment throughout treatment.[5] *Note:* assessment in patients with colostomy is a challenge and depends on volume of stool (see Appendix A).

❖ Teach the patient the dose and schedule of prescribed antidiarrheal medication, monitor compliance, and evaluate their effectiveness.[5] See Table 12-2.

TABLE 12-2
Antidiarrheal Agents[16,34]

Drug	Dose and Frequency
Loperamide (standard dose)	4 mg (2 [2mg] capsules) after the first loose stool, followed by 2 mg (1 capsule) after each subsequent loose stool; maximum dose 16mg/day. *Note: This dosage and schedule is not recommended for irinotecan containing regimens.*
Loperamide (irinotecan dose)	4 mg (2 [2mg] capsules) at the first change in bowel habits, followed by 2 mg (1 capsule) every 2 hours until diarrhea free for 12 hours; Take a 4-mg dose (2 [2-mg] capsules) every 4 hours during the night.
Diphenoxylate hydrochloride with atropine sulfate	5 mg PO QID initially. Titrate up or down to response. Discontinue if not effective in 48 hours, if blood is noted in stool, or if fever is present.
Deodorized tincture of Opium	0.3 to 1 mL QID. Maximum dose of 6 mL/day, or 5–10 drops (0.6 mL) after each stool to a maximum of 6 doses/day.
Octreotide acetate	Standard dose: 100 μg BID or 150 μg TID SQ
	High dose: 1,500 μg TID SQ. Titrate to response (range 450–1,500 μg/day)
Octreotide LAR Depot	20 or 30 mg IM q 4 weeks under investigation
Glutamine	10 g PO TID for 4–5 days starting the evening before or day of therapy and continuing for 3–4 days after treatment under investigation.
Kaopectate	60–120 mL (regular) or 45–90 mL (concentrated) solution PO after each loose stool, for a maximum duration of 48 hours
Paregoric	0.3–1 mL. Mix with water. Titrate dose from 1–4 times per day.

* Treatments vary based on the underlying cause and include pharmacologic, dietary modifications, and alterations in treatment dose.
* Evaluate the effectiveness of the antidiarrheal regimen and alter as appropriate
* Monitor electrolyte balance, especially potassium and sodium
* Advise the patient to document their elimination pattern: precipitating factors, onset of diarrhea, number of episodes, duration of diarrhea, and description of stools (color, consistency, etc.); report abnormalities to the physician or nurse[5]
* Teach the patient about dietary and fluid recommendations. Table 12-3.[5]
* Teach the patient about perianal and stomal skin care; assess effectiveness[5]
* Consider the need for delay or dose modifications with the physician making adjustments according to the manufacturer's or protocol's recommendations
* Report to the physician or nurse any changes in the abdomen and/or stool pattern especially in the first cycle of treatment

❖ Alopecia

Nursing Interventions:

* Educate the patient about the expected timing of hair loss, usually 10 to 21 days after the initiation of treatment

TABLE 12–3
Diarrhea and Dietary Suggestions[5,16]

Foods and liquids to encourage:

a. Bland, easily digested foods, such as the BRAT diet: *b*ananas, white *r*ice, *a*pplesauce, *t*oast; gelatins, yogurt, sherbet; cooked foods at room temperature

b. Small frequent meals

c. Water, carbohydrate-electrolyte beverages, clear broth, diluted fruit juice: Increase liquid intake to 2 to 3 quarts per day total.

d. Foods that contain salt and potassium

e. Such foods as boiled or baked potatoes without the skin, pasta, skinless baked or broiled chicken and fish, canned fruit, well cooked vegetables, and crackers: Increase these types of foods once diarrhea resolves.

Foods and liquids to avoid:

a. Foods that are raw or high in fiber or roughage, such as whole-grain breads and cereals, popcorn, fresh fruit, dried beans, raw vegetables (corn, pumpkin, broccoli, cauliflower, cabbage), nuts

b. Foods that are rich, seasoned, spicy, fatty, greasy, or very hot

c. Milk products and milk, alcohol, caffeinated and very hot beverages

---

❖ Reinforce that hair loss is temporary, that it may involve thinning of body hair, and that hair will regrow at completion of the treatment plan

❖ Encourage the patient to purchase head coverings—for example, wigs, caps, scarves, bandanas—prior to hair loss, and to wear them year-round

- ❖ Refer patient to "Look Good Feel Better" program
- ❖ Educate the patient to avoid excessive or harsh hair treatments
- ❖ Encourage the patient to verbalize his or her feelings about hair loss, and provide emotional support
- ❖ Radiotherapy to the pelvis will cause permanent loss of pubic hair.

❖ Alteration in sexual function

Nursing Interventions:

- ❖ Initiate a trusting relationship to establish open lines of communication
- ❖ Conduct a baseline sexual history
- ❖ Assess and review with the patient and significant other the potential causes in sexual dysfunction that may occur because of the disease and the treatment[6]
  1. Surgical removal of ovaries and/or uterus, nerve damage or scar tissue
  2. Radiation and/or chemotherapy damage to ovaries or testes. Effects may include infertility, inability to achieve or sustain an erection, or retrograde ejaculation.
  3. Anxiety and/or depression may decrease interest in sexual activity.
- ❖ Prior to treatment, encourage sperm banking or ova harvesting and banking
- ❖ Suggest prevention measures, e.g., dilators 3 times/week to prevent vaginal scarring from radiation therapy

> ❖ Discuss behavioral strategies to minimize the impact of the dysfunction[6]
>> 1. Create a sensual environment
>> 2. Explore alternative forms of sexual expression
>> 3. Use mechanical devices or medications to aid erections
>> 4. Use vaginal lubricants or hormone creams
> ❖ Refer the patient and significant other for reproductive counseling, as appropriate
> ❖ Encourage open lines of communication between patient and partner

Nursing Management Issues with Specific Agents

❖ Information on 5-FU and leucovorin can be found in Chapter 9.

Irinotecan (CPT-11)

❖ Recommended regimens:[7]

> ❖ First-line therapy:
>> 1. Irinotecan 125 mg/m^2 IV over 90* minutes, 5-fluorouracil (5-FU) 500 mg/m^2 IV push, leucovorin (LV) 20 mg/m^2 IV push q week x 4 every 6 weeks (bolus IFL)
>> 2. Irinotecan 180 mg/m^2 IV over 90* minutes, LV 200 mg/m^2 IV over 2 hours, 5-FU 400mg/m^2 IV bolus, followed by 5-FU 600 mg/m^2 continuous IV infusion over 22 hours days 1 and 2 every 2 weeks (Infusional IFL)

  3. Irinotecan 180mg/m^2 IV over 90 minutes, LV
     200 mg/m^2 IV over 2 hours, 5-FU 400 mg/m^2
     IV bolus, followed by 5-FU 2.4 to 3 gms
     continuous IV infusion over 46 hours every
     2 weeks (FOLFIRI, investigational regimen)[8]

❖ Second line therapy:[7]

  1. Irinotecan 125 mg/m^2 IV over 90* minutes q
     week x 4 every 6 weeks
  2. Irinotecan 350 mg/m^2 IV over 90* minutes
     q3 weeks

❖ Special considerations: Should not be administered in patients with bilirubin >2.0 mg/dL,
  Gilbert's disease, or transaminase >3 × upper
  limit of normal without liver metastasis. Close
  monitoring is recommended for patients with a
  performance status ≥2, previously treated with
  pelvic/abdominal radiotherapy, and the elderly
  with comorbid conditions.[7]

❖ Common toxicities: cholinergic syndrome, late-
  onset diarrhea, neutropenia, nausea, vomiting,
  and hair loss[7]

❖ Reported but less common toxicities: mucositis
  and febrile neutropenia.[7]

---

*Note: Though not recommended by the manufacturer, irinotecan has been
administered over 30 minutes without increase in toxicity[9] and is being
investigated in a schedule of 2 weeks of treatment followed by 1 week off
every 3 weeks.[10]

❖ Cholinergic syndrome

  ❖ Signs and symptoms: may include one or any combination of the following: rhinorrhea, nasal congestion, lacrimation, salivation, diaphoresis, flushing, intestinal cramping, diarrhea, nausea, and vomiting[11]

  ❖ Characteristics: usually occurs during or shortly after administration of irinotecan, is often transient, and infrequently severe

  ❖ Treatment (including prophylaxis): intravenous or subcutaneous atropine at a dose of 0.25 mg to 1.0 mg; symptoms resolve within 10 minutes.[7,12]

❖ Late-onset diarrhea

  ❖ Signs and symptoms: change in usual bowel habits, such as watery stools, poorly formed or loose stools, an increase in number of bowel movements compared with usual number, or late abdominal cramping with or without diarrhea

  ❖ Characteristics: occur more than 24 hours after irinotecan administration; can be life threatening if prolonged, resulting in dehydration, electrolyte imbalance, or sepsis; variation in onset based on irinotecan schedule.[7,13]

	CPT-11 Weekly	CPT-11 Every 3 weeks	IFL Combination
Median time to onset	~11 days	~5 days	~7 days
Duration	~3 days	~9 days	~2–4 days

❖ Treatment:

1. Intensive dose of loperamide as per special instructions:[7]

   a. At the first sign of diarrhea, take 4 mg (2 [2-mg] capsules) of loperamide, then 2 mg (1 capsule) every 2 hours until free of diarrhea for at least 12 hours. Take a 4-mg dose (2 [2-mg] capsules) every 4 hours during the night. (*Note:* this dose exceeds the usual loperamide dose.)

2. Upon failure with loperamide, additional options such as lomotil, tincture of opium, octreotide, and glutamine, used with anecdotal success, are noted in Table 12-2.[5,16]

3. Nontraditional methods are also being explored:

   a. A recent report suggests a specific dietary intervention of at least 100 mg sugar and 2 gms of sodium can impact the incidence of severe diarrhea.[14] A 16% decrease in severe diarrhea and a 7% reduction in hospitalization was reported. Approximately 93% of chemotherapy doses were associated with no evidence of severe diarrhea.[14] Sugar and sodium recipe involves drinking Koolaid (unsweetened) mixed with 2 cups of sugar in 2 quarts of water or jello-tea (one package of jello mixed in warm/hot water) **plus** one can Campbell's soup (not low-salt variety) **or** 2 bouillon cubes dissolved in water. Drink Koolaid and soup regimen 3 consecutive days (day of infusion + 2 days after). (Oral communication, June 14, 2002, Dr. Edith Mitchell)

   b. Thalidomide, 400 mg at bedtime, reportedly may also decrease the incidence of irinotecan-induced severe diarrhea.[15] Research is ongoing.

  4. Patients should notify nurse or physician immediately for diarrhea occurring for the first time, inability to control diarrhea within 24 hours, black or bloody stools, signs of dehydration, severe nausea and/or vomiting preventing oral intake of fluids, fever >100.5°F, and/or signs of infection.[7]

❖ Dose delay and/or reductions[7]

  1. The manufacturer recommends dose delays and/or reductions based on the severity and duration of diarrhea.[7]

  2. If diarrhea persists within 24 hours of next scheduled dosage, therapy should be delayed until diarrhea resolves without antidiarrheal medication.[7]

  3. Manufacturer's recommendations for dose adjustments of both irinotecan and 5-FU in the combination irinotecan, 5-FU, plus leucovorin regimen are noted in Tables 12-4 and 12-5.[7]

TABLE 12-4
Manufacturer's Dose Adjustment Recommendations for Irinotecan Induced Diarrhea

Diarrhea NCI CTC Grade Version 1.0	Combination therapy During a Cycle of Therapy	At the Start of Subsequent Cycles of Therapy (Relative to Starting Dose Used in Previous Cycle)
1 (2–3 stools/day > baseline)	Delay dose until resolved to baseline, then give same dose	Maintain dose level
2 (4–6 stools/day > baseline)	Omit dose until resolved to baseline, then ↓ 1 dose level	Maintain dose level
3 (7–9 stools/day > baseline)	Omit dose until resolved to baseline then ↓ 1 dose level	↓ 1 dose level
4 (≥10 stools/day > baseline)	Omit dose until resolved to baseline then ↓ 2 dose level	↓ 2 dose level

TABLE 12-5
Manufacturer's Recommended Dose Levels

Drug	Starting Dose and Modified Dose Levels (mg/m^2)		
Regimen 1 Bolus IFL Weekly treatment × 4 q 6 weeks	Starting Dose	Dose Level –1	Dose Level –2
Irinotecan	125	100	75
Leucovorin	20	20	20
5-FU	500	400	300
Regimen 2 Infusional IFL Treatment q 2 weeks	Starting Dose	Dose Level –1	Dose Level –2
Irinotecan	180	150	120
Leucovorin	200	200	200
5-FU bolus dose	400	320	240
5-FU infusional dose	600	480	360

4. Manufacturer's recommendations for dose adjustments for single agent irinotecan are noted in Table 12-6.[7]

❖ Monitoring

1. Carefully monitor patients and administer appropriate supportive therapies, e.g., IV fluids, antibiotics, if they develop dehydration, ileus, fever, or severe neutropenia[7]

❖ Diet

1. Dietary modifications, as noted in Table 12-3, may be helpful.

❖ Neutropenia

❖ Signs and symptoms: decrease in circulating neutrophil count to less than 1000/uL

❖ Characteristics: the onset of neutropenia varies based on the irinotecan schedule.[13]

	CPT-11 Weekly	CPT-11 Every 3 weeks	IFL Combination
Median time to nadir	~21 days	~8 days	~14 days
Duration	~7–14 days	~7–9 days	~9 days

❖ Treatment: dose delay and reductions are recommended based on the severity of the neutropenia. Specific recommendations for combination IFL therapy are noted in Table 12-7:[7]

1. With the combination regimen, both irinotecan and 5-FU must be reduced if appropriate. LV does not change. See Table 12-5 above for specific doses (mg/m^2).

TABLE 12-6 Manufacturer's Dose Adjustment Recommendations for Irinotecan-Induced Diarrhea

	Single Agent Irinotecan	At the Start of Subsequent Cycles of Therapy (Relative to Starting Dose Used in Previous Cycle)	
Diarrhea NCI CTC Grade Version 1.0	During a Cycle of Therapy	Weekly	Once Every 3 Weeks
1 (2–3 stools/day > baseline)	Maintain dose	Maintain dose level	Maintain dose level
2 (4–6 stools/day > baseline)	↓ 25 mg/m²	Maintain dose level	Maintain dose level
3 (7–9 stools/day > baseline)	Omit dose until resolved ≤ grade 2 then ↓ 25 mg/m²	↓ 25 mg/m²	↓ 50mg/m²
4 (≥10 stools/day > baseline)	Omit dose until resolved ≤ grade 2 then ↓ 50 mg/m²	↓ 50mg/m²	↓ 50mg/m²

TABLE 12–7
Manufacturer's Dose Adjustment Recommendations for Irinotecan-Induced Neutiopenia

Neutropenia NCI CTC Grade Version 1.0	Combination therapy During a Cycle of Therapy	At the Start of Subsequent Cycles of Therapy (Relative to Starting Dose Used in Previous Cycle)
1 (1500 to 1999/mm³)	Maintain dose level	Maintain dose level
2 (1000 to 1499/mm³)	↓ 1 dose level	Maintain dose level
3 (500 to 999/mm³)	Omit dose until resolved ≤ grade 2 then ↓ 1 dose level	↓ 1 dose level
4 (<500/mm³)	Omit dose until resolved ≤ grade 2 then ↓ 2 dose levels	↓ 2 dose levels

    2. Manufacturer's recommendation for dose reduction of single agent irinotecan is noted in Table 12-8:[7]

❖ Additional key management considerations:

    1. Consider initial dose modifications in patients previously treated with pelvic or abdominal radiation therapy, elderly with comorbid conditions, patients with a performance status of 2, or who have increased bilirubin levels (range 1 to 2 mg/dL)[7]

    2. Avoid magnesium-containing medications which may increase diarrhea[7]

    3. ASCO does not recommend standard use of growth factors in this population, but this may be considered in individual patients.[2]

❖ Nausea and vomiting

    ❖ Signs and Symptoms: acute or delayed incidence

    ❖ Characteristics: moderately emetogenic

    ❖ Treatment: Premedicate at least 30 minutes before infusion with dexamethasone (10–20 mg IV) plus an antiemetic agent.[7] Antiemetogenic guidelines for moderate emetogenic potential agents suggest the use of a 5-hydroxytryptamine type 3 [5-HT$_3$] blocker.[16] See Table 12-1.

    ❖ Prochlorperazine is recommended for delayed nausea and/or vomiting, but not on the same day as irinotecan administration, because of an increased frequency of akathesia.[7]

TABLE 12-8 Manufacturer's Dose Adjustment Recommendations for Irinotecan-Induced Neutropenia

Neutropenia NCI CTC Grade Version 1.0	Single Agent Irinotecan During a Cycle of Therapy	At the Start of Subsequent Cycles of Therapy (Relative to Starting Dose Used in Previous Cycle)	
		Weekly	Once Every 3 Weeks
1 (1500 to 1999/mm^3)	Maintain dose	Maintain dose level	Maintain dose level
2 (1000 to 1499/mm^3)	↓ 25 mg/m^2	Maintain dose level	Maintain dose level
3 (500 to 999/mm^3)	Omit dose until resolved ≤ grade 2 then ↓ 25 mg/m^2	↓ 25 mg/m^2	↓ 50 mg/m^2
4 (<500/mm^3)	Omit dose until resolved ≤ grade 2 then ↓ 50 mg/m^2	↓ 50 mg/m^2	↓ 50 mg/m^2

❖ Metoclopramide is not recommended as an antiemetic as it may contribute to diarrhea.

❖ Special programs/materials:

❖ Patient education brochures, such as "Your Guide to Treatment" and " Everyday Advice" provide both information about irinotecan-based therapy and a diary for toxicity reporting. These brochures are available free of charge from Pharmacia Oncology.

❖ A complete dosing and dose modification guide is available at <u>www.pharmaciaoncology.com/products.asp?Cttypes=7&Ptype=2</u>.

Capecitabine

❖ Recommended regimen:

❖ 1250 mg/m^2 orally twice daily (BID) for 2 weeks followed by a 1-week rest period every 3 weeks. Doses should be taken approximately 12 hours apart within 30 minutes after the end of a meal. Tablets should be swallowed with a full glass of water.[17] *Note:* though a lower starting dose of 1000 mg/m^2 BID is common in clinical practice, this dose has not been validated for efficacy.

❖ An electronic dosing guide for handheld computers is downloadable from <u>www.xeloda.com/web/colorectal/indexasp?pgdsp=116</u>.

❖ Common toxicities: palmar-plantar erythrodysesthesia (hand and foot syndrome), diarrhea, fatigue, abdominal pain, dermatitis, nausea, vomiting, anorexia, and stomatitis[17]

❖ Reported but less common toxicities: anemia, transient hyperbilirubinemia, hair loss, and bone marrow suppression[17]

❖ Special considerations:[17]

  ❖ Monitor bilirubin before and throughout therapy; dose modifications are recommended for hyperbilirubinemia.

  ❖ Contraindicated in patients with severe renal impairment.[17] Patients with mild renal impairment should be closely monitored. Patients with moderate impairment (30–50 mL/min) would be treated at 950 mg/m^2 BID (75% of the recommended starting dose) in conjunction with careful monitoring.[17]

❖ Drug interactions: LV may increase the incidence and severity of gastrointestinal toxicity.[17] Maalox, or other antacids containing magnesium- and aluminum-hydroxides, may affect the absorption of capecitabine.[17] Patients taking warfarin or coumarin-derivative anticoagulants may have altered coagulation parameters and/or bleeding. Close monitoring of PT or INR is recommended. Phenytoin taken concomitantly may result in abnormal phenytoin levels.[17]

❖ Diarrhea

  ❖ Signs and symptoms: increase in the number of stools per day over baseline

  ❖ Characteristics: time to first occurrence of grade 2 to 4 diarrhea is 34 days.[17]

* ❖ Treatment: Antidiarrheal medications according to physician preference; withhold therapy for toxicity ≥ grade 2.[17] See Table 12-2 for antidiarrheal medications.
* ❖ Special considerations: Patients > 80 years old experience a greater incidence of severe gastrointestinal side effects; therefore, caution should be exercised in the older patient.[17] Registration trials excluded patients with performance status 2 (see Appendix B for definitions) so no data is available on how this group will tolerate capecitabine.[17]

❖ Hand and foot syndrome (HFS) also called Palmar-plantar erythrodysesthesia (PPE)

* ❖ Signs and symptoms:
  1. Early symptoms: dry furrowed skin, which then turns mildly erythemic, with tingling sensation or numbness, painless swelling, tenderness, rash or dry/itchy skin on the palms of the hands and soles of the feet[17,18]
  2. Later symptoms: progressively worse—painful erythema, swelling, discomfort with activities of daily living (grade 2) to desquamation, ulceration, blistering, or severe pain (grade 3)[17]
* ❖ Treatment: stop therapy at grade 2 symptoms until HFS has resolved (may take 3 to 7 days).[17] Future dose recommendations are based on the severity and frequency as recommended by the manufacturer.[17,18]

1. Symptomatic/prophylactic treatment: emollient lotions or creams containing lanolin to keep skin hydrated; if more severe, soak hands in cool to tepid water for 10 minutes then apply petroleum jelly to wet skin.[17,18] Vitamin B6, celecoxib, cotton gloves, ice packs, and/or decreasing pressure to the palms and soles, e.g., avoid tight fitting shoes/clothes, may be used.[16]

   a. Pyridoxine (Vitamin B6) Patients who receive 200 mg/d derived a greater benefit than those who received less.[19] Anecdotally, dosing ranges from 50 to 150 mg/day for prophylaxis; 100 to 300 mg/day for treatment.

   b. Celebrex 200 mg PO BID has demonstrated effects in reducing HFS and diarrhea, possibly through an anti-inflammatory mechanism.[20]

   c. Lac-Hydrin anecdotally appears to minimize HFS; prophylactic use may provide maximum benefit. Emollients minimize the dryness that precedes HFS, but are messy.

2. Patient must recognize any signs of progression and report changes to the physician and/or nurse.[18]

3. A higher percentage of patients 70 to 79 years of age developed severe HFS; therefore, caution should be exercised in treating the older patient.[17]

❖ Nausea and vomiting

❖ Signs and symptoms: acute or delayed; frequent toxicity

❖ Characteristics: mildly emetogenic

❖ Treatment: Antiemetic medications according to physician preference for mildly emetogenic agents. Premedicate and continue for 24 hours. Fluid and electrolyte replacement as necessary.[18] See Table 12-1 for Antiemetic Agents.

❖ Miscellaneous Issues:

❖ The *key* intervention is to hold doses of capecitabine for moderate to severe toxicity until the toxicity has resolved.[18]

❖ Doses withheld during treatment interruptions are not replaced, and once the dose has been decreased, it should not be increased at a later cycle. Doses are taken days 1–14 so if doses are held on days 8–9, those are not made up, but treatment resumes for days 10–14.[17]

❖ Compliance is a major concern with oral chemotherapy agents, both in terms of taking the medication as ordered and stopping it for toxicity. Educating the patient and family about the treatment plan, potential side effects, and self-care measures is extremely important. Encourage patients to call to report first appearance of side effect, so teaching can be reinforced about holding and calibrating future doses. Toughing out toxicity will not benefit the patient.

❖ The following stopping rules are recommended:[17]

1. *Diarrhea:* an increase of 4 or more stools each day or any diarrhea at night
2. *Vomiting:* two or more episodes in a 24-hour time period
3. *Nausea:* loss of appetite or a significant decrease in the amount of food eaten each day
4. *Stomatitis:* painful redness, swelling, or sores in the mouth or tongue
5. *Hand and foot syndrome:* painful swelling or redness of hands and/or feet or any change that limits activities of daily living
6. *Fever or infection:* temperature of ≥100.5°F or other sign of infection

❖ Subsequent doses are based on the severity and the frequency of the toxicity as noted Table 12-9:[17]

❖ Special Programs/Materials

❖ The "Xtra" (Xeloda Therapy Reinforcement Access) program provides patients with extra support and education materials. More information about this program can be obtained by calling (877) XTRA-4-US (1-877-987-2487).[17]

❖ "Frankly Speaking about Colorectal Cancer" is an education kit created for patients and families. It is available free of charge from The Wellness Community (1-888-793-WELL).

TABLE 12-9
Manufacturer's Dose Adjustment Recommendations

National Cancer Institute of Canada Common Toxicity Criteria	Capecitabine Recommended Dose Modifications		
	Capecitabine dose changes during current treatment period	*Capecitabine dose adjustments for resumption of treatment*	
Grade 1	100% of starting dose	100% of starting dose	
Grade 2	Start symptomatic treatment where possible		
1st appearance	Interrupt until resolved (grade 0–1)	100% of starting dose	
2nd appearance	Interrupt until resolved (grade 0–1)	75% of starting dose	
3rd appearance	Interrupt until resolved (grade 0–1)	50% of starting dose	
4th appearance	Discontinue permanently		

(continued)

TABLE 12-9
Manufacturer's Dose Adjustment Recommendations (continued)

National Cancer Institute of Canada Common Toxicity Criteria	Capecitabine Recommended Dose Modifications	
	Capecitabine dose changes during current treatment period	Capecitabine dose adjustments for resumption of treatment
Grade 3	Start symptomatic treatment where possible	
1st appearance	Interrupt until resolved (grade 0–1)	75% of starting dose
2nd appearance	Interrupt until resolved (grade 0–1)	50% of starting dose
3rd appearance	Discontinue permanently	
Grade 4		
1st appearance	Discontinue permanently or interrupt until resolved (grade 0–1)	Reduce to 50%

❖ Reimbursement hotline: (800) 443–6676. Reimbursement is an issue for some patient populations. Medicare will cover 80% of capecitabine. The patient or secondary insurance is responsible for the remaining 20% plus any deductibles. Patients with other insurance or prescription plans may have the same requirements. This can be problematic when filling the prescription at the local pharmacy.[17]

Oxaliplatin

❖ Recommended regimen

❖ Second-line therapy (FDA approved regimen)

1. Oxaliplatin 85 mg/m^2 IV over 2–6 hours on day 1, LV 200 mg/m^2 IV over 2 hours, 5-FU 400 mg/m^2 IV bolus followed by 5-FU 600 mg/m^2 continuous intravenous infusion over 22 hours on days 1 and 2 every 2 weeks (FOLFOX 4)[21,22]

❖ Regimens in the literature:[11]

1. Oxaliplatin 85 mg/m^2 IV over 2–6 hours, LV 200 mg/m^2 IV over 2 hours, 5-FU 400 mg/m^2 IV bolus followed by 5-FU 2.4 to 3 gm/m^2 continuous intravenous infusion over 46 hours every 2 weeks (FOLFOX 6)[8] (note there are at least 9 different FOLFOX regimens in the literature)

2. Oxaliplatin 85 mg/m² IV over 2–6 hours every 2 weeks
3. Oxaliplatin 130 mg/m² IV over 2–6 hours every 3 weeks

❖ Other regimens involve the various 5-FU and LV schedules.[11]

❖ Common toxicities: cold-induced peripheral sensory neuropathy, acute laryngopharyngeal dysesthesia, nausea, vomiting, muscle cramping, diarrhea, stomatitis, neutropenia, anemia, thrombocytopenia, and fatigue[11,21,22]

❖ Reported but less common toxicities: anaphylactic-like reactions, allergic reactions, pulmonary fibrosis, hand and foot syndrome, alopecia, and elevated hepatic enzymes[11,21,22]

❖ *Note:* Unlike other platinum agents, oxaliplatin is not associated with nephro- or ototoxicity; therefore, intravenous prehydration is not required.[22]

❖ *Note:* When given in combination with 5-FU, the specific 5-FU regimen greatly influences the toxicity profile.[11]

❖ Peripheral sensory neuropathy

❖ Signs and symptoms: numbness and tingling in the perioral area, throat fingers and/or toes, with distal dysesthesias.[11] Jaw pain, abnormal tongue sensations, dysarthrea, eye pain, and chest pressure also reported.[22]

❖ Characteristics: cold-induced; acute and chronic neuropathy; onset within hours to days, resolves before the next dose of oxaliplatin in earlier cycles, but tends to last longer with subsequent cycles. Neurologic toxicity is cumulative but reversible over time.[11,22]

❖ Treatment: No current treatment is recommended to prevent neurotoxicity. Acute neurotoxicity can be reduced through education (see recommendation #3). Chronic neurotoxicity is expected with continued dosing, but treatment should be discontinued before severe impairment occurs.[11]

1. Investigational approaches include administration of calcium gluconate and magnesium chloride infusions, neurontin, phenytoin, capsaicin cream, EMLA cream, and topical lidocaine.[23,24,25]

    a. Calcium 1 gm and magnesium 1 gm IV before and after oxaliplatin infusions has demonstrated effects in reducing incidence and intensity of acute neurosensory symptoms and possibly chronic neutrotoxicity.[23]

    b. Neurontin (gabapentin) at doses of 100 mg/BID, with doses increased 100mg/day as needed if symptoms did not disappear, provided complete relief of neurologic toxicity. When gabapentin was stopped the symptoms returned; when it was restarted, the symptoms again resolved.[25]

2. Prior to each dose of oxaliplatin, assess the patient for signs of neurologic toxicity (e.g., ability to pick up small objects, write their name, ability to walk without difficulties).[11,22]

3. Educate patients to stay away from cold especially within the first 48 to 96 hours of treatment; for example, avoid holding (and drinking) cold beverages or foods; avoid use of ice, avoid putting hands into the refrigerator or freezer; avoid cold showers or baths; avoid going outside in cold weather or decreasing temperature of air conditioning.[11]

❖ Acute laryngopharyngeal dysesthesia

 ❖ Signs and symptoms: sensation of tightness in the throat; choking sensation, subjective feeling of dyspnea and/or dysphagia, with accompanying anxiety[11]

 ❖ Characteristics: cold-induced; transient, onset within hours of infusion reported in 1–2% of patients[22]

 ❖ Treatment:

1. Treatment for immediate complaints: Rule out airway obstruction; may assess blood gases, though they are usually normal; there are no recommended interventions, because it often resolves spontaneously. Anxiolytics may be administered.[24]

2. Preventative measures: **Do not** use ice chips to prevent mucositis; avoid drinking cold

beverages during or within several hours to days after treatment.[11] Oxaliplatin infusion can be lengthened to 6 hours, which will reduce the incidence. Patients need to be aware of this potential side effect as it is a frightening sensation.[11] Anxiolytics may be administered prophylactically before subsequent treatments.[23]

3. A unique grading scale, developed for the clinical trials, provides criteria for assessing the intensity, duration, and functional status for the patient receiving oxaliplatin (Table 12-10).

❖ Nausea and vomiting

  ❖ Signs and symptoms: acute or delayed incidence
  ❖ Characteristics: moderately emetogenic
  ❖ Treatment: Premedicate at least 30 minutes before infusion with a 5-hydroxytryptamine type 3 (5-HT$_3$) blocker of choice and dexamethasone.[11] See Table 12-1 for Antiemetic Agents.

❖ Thrombocytopenia

  ❖ Signs and symptoms: mild to moderate decrease in platelet count
  ❖ Characteristics: In some patients, platelet count stabilizes at a moderately low level (between approximately 75,000 to 100,000/uL).[11]
  ❖ Treatment: Monitor platelet count at baseline and throughout therapy. Hold doses as recommended by manufacturer or per clinical trial for severity of thrombocytopenia.[11]

TABLE 12-10
Oxaliplatin Specific Neurologic Toxicity Scale For Clinical Trials[22,33]

Toxicity	Symptoms
Severity	
Peripheral-Sensory Neuropathy	
Grade 1 (mild)	Paresthesias and/or dysesthesias of limited duration; no interference with function; resolution before next cycle of therapy
Grade 2 (moderate)	Paresthesias and/or dysesthesias lasting in-between cycles of therapy; interfers with function but not daily activities
Grade 3 (severe)	Paresthesias and/or dysesthesias lasting in-between cycles of therapy; alteration in activities of daily living with functional impairment; pain
Grade 4 (life-threatening)	Disabling or life-threatening paresthesias and/or dysesthesias
Laryngeal-Dysesthesias	
Mild	No description available
Moderate	No description available
Severe	No description available

❖ Neutropenia

  ❖ Signs and symptoms: decrease in circulating
    neutrophil count of less than 1000/uL
  ❖ Characteristics: the onset of neutropenia varies
    based on the chemotherapy regimen.
  ❖ Treatment: Dose delay and reductions are rec-
    ommended in the clinical trial and are based on
    the severity of the neutropenia. Per ASCO
    guidelines, standard use of growth factors in
    this population is not recommended, but may
    be considered in individual patients.[2]

❖ Anaphylactic-like/allergic/hypersensitivity reactions

  ❖ Signs and symptoms: rash, shortness of breath,
    dizziness, bronchospasm, rigors, chills,
    hypotension, fever, confusion urticaria, ery-
    thema, and pruritus[22]
  ❖ Characteristics: may occur during or within
    hours after the infusion; median time to
    reaction was 6 doses (range 2–20).[25] Incidence
    approximately 3%[22]
  ❖ Treatment:

    1. Immediate reaction: Stop the drug, notify
       physician; standard treatment for anaphy-
       latic reactions usually includes epinephrine
       1:1000, hydrocortisone, and diphenhy-
       dramine. Treat rigors with meperidine. Treat
       fever symptomatically.
    2. Prophylactic measures for future treatments:
       Discuss future administration with physician.
       In one study, dexamethasone 20 mg, cimeti-

dine 300mg, acetaminophen 650 mg, and diphenhydramine 25mg, in addition to a prolonged infusion time, allowed for continuation of therapy.[26]

❖ Muscle cramping[24]

  ❖ Signs and symptoms: involuntary contraction of a muscle primarily in the hand or forearm
  ❖ Characteristics: often associated with cold
  ❖ Treatment: Often resolves spontaneously; warmth to the affected area can provide at least some relief.

❖ Diarrhea

  ❖ Signs and symptoms: increase in the number of stools per day over baseline
  ❖ Characteristics: often mild, but frequency increases when combined with 5-FU and leucovorin.
  ❖ Treatment: Antidiarrheal medications and dose adjustments according to physician preference or protocol outline; see Table 12-2 for Antidiarrheal Medications.

❖ Stomatitis

  ❖ Signs and symptoms: erythema potentially progressing to pain and ulceration
  ❖ Characteristics: onset varies with specific chemotherapy regimen; common side effect
  ❖ Treatment: **Do not** recommend cryotherapy. Preventive measures, topical protective agents, antibiotics, pain medications if symptoms worsen, and soft or liquid foods high in protein

are recommended. Dose delay or reductions may be appropriate based on physician discretion and/or the protocol.

Cetuximab (C225)

❖ Recommended regimen: (investigational in the treatment of colorectal cancer)

  ❖ Test dose—20 mg/10 mL IV over 10 minutes—followed by an observation period of 30 minutes. If no reaction, loading dose follows at 400 mg/m^2 (less the amount of the test dose) IV over 120 minutes, followed by weekly doses of 250 mg/m^2 IV over 60 minutes.[27] *Note:* When given with chemotherapy, the additional agent will greatly influence the side effect profile.[28]

❖ Common toxicities: allergic reactions, skin reactions, asthenia, fever, nausea, and elevated SGPT[28]

❖ Allergic reactions

  ❖ Signs and symptoms: generalized itching, nausea, chest tightness, crampy abdominal pain, anxiety, dizziness, chills, flushed appearance, edema, urticaria, and rarely anaphylactic reactions[28]

  ❖ Characteristics: All reactions thus far have occurred only during the test dose. Usually mild.[28]

  ❖ Treatment: Stop drug immediately, notify physician; standard treatment for anaphylactic reactions usually includes epinephrine 1:1000, hydrocortisone, and diphenhydramine. For mild reactions, prophylactic antihistamine treatment and prolonged infusion time allowed for continuation of therapy.[28]

❖ Acne-like rash

  ❖ Signs and symptoms: rash, folliculitis, and maculopapular lesions especially on the face, upper chest and back[28]

  ❖ Characteristics: Common, occurs in about 80% of patients; onset during first 2 weeks of treatment and may diminish as treatment continues. Usually mild, but it may be severe. Reversible within 4-8 weeks once the drug is discontinued.[28]

  ❖ Treatment: Topical or systemic oral antibiotics, topical hydrocortisone, or topical retinoids have been given without clear improvement.[28] Cosmetic recommendations and patient education are important to temper the emotional impact of this visible toxicity.

Thalidomide

❖ Recommended regimen: (investigational in the treatment of colorectal cancer)

  ❖ 200–400 mg/day orally[15,29,30]

❖ Common toxicities: teratogenicity, neurologic toxicities (sedation, peripheral neuropathy, and constipation), hypotension, and peripheral edema[29,30]

❖ Reported but less common toxicities: thromboembolic events, neutropenia, and skin rashes[29]

❖ Special Consideration: S.T.E.P.S. (System for Thalidomide Education and Prescribing Safety). All prescribers, pharmacists, and patients must be registered and are educated about thalidomide and its teratogenicity. The program has very specific details about birth control measures:[29,30]

 ❖ Women of childbearing age must have a negative pregnancy test each month of treatment and use two forms of birth control; men are required to use a latex condom during sexual intercourse with women of childbearing potential.

❖ Sedation
 ❖ Signs and symptoms: drowsiness, hangover, daytime sleepiness, dizziness, fatigue, weakness, incoordination, shakiness, mood changes, confusion, and blurred vision[30]
 ❖ Characteristics: may moderate after 2 to 4 weeks of therapy, increased risk in elderly[30]
 ❖ Treatment: Dose reduction is often effective. Taking prescribed dose at bedtime is also a recommendation.[29] Teach patients to avoid other medications that cause sedation, such as alcoholic beverages, narcotics, antidepressants, and anxiolytics.[30]

❖ Peripheral neuropathy
 ❖ Signs and symptoms: numbness and tingling of the hands and feet
 ❖ Characteristics: similar in mechanism to that caused by the taxanes, vincristine, and cisplatin.[30] Often mild but can progress in severity.

* Treatment: Assess neurologic status at each visit; discontinuation of therapy may be required.[30]

❖ Constipation
  * Signs and symptoms: absence of stool for 2 days
  * Characteristics: usually mild
  * Treatment: Prevention is key—increased fluid intake, increased dietary fiber, regular exercise, and a bowel regimen with stool softeners, mild laxatives, or bulk agents (e.g., psyllium), then adjusted based on effectiveness.[30]

❖ Miscellaneous toxicities:
  * Bedtime dosing may alleviate daytime hypotension. Peripheral edema usually does not require intervention, but diuretics may be prescribed as needed.[30]

Bevacizumab

❖ Recommended regimen: (investigational in the treatment of colorectal cancer)
  * 5 mg/kg to 10mg/kg IV over 90 minutes every 2 weeks. May slowly decrease infusion time to 60 then 30 minutes if tolerated.[31]

❖ Common Toxicities: hypersensitivity reactions, acute hypertension, thrombosis, bleeding and headache

❖ Hypersensitivity reaction
  * Signs and symptoms: fever, rigors, chills, and rash
  * Characteristics: May occur during infusion

* Treatment: Stop the infusion, notify physician; standard treatment for anaphylatic reactions usually includes epinephrine 1:1000, hydrocortisone, and diphenhydramine; may also require oxygen and IV fluids. Treat fever symptomatically. Treat rigors with meperidine. For mild reactions, prophylactic diphenhydramine 25 mg IV and rantidine 50 mg IV and prolonged infusion time may allow for continuation of therapy.[31]

* Hypertension
  * Signs and symptoms: sudden elevation in blood pressure
  * Treatment: Monitor blood pressure during treatment, symptomatic measures as per physician. Acute or uncontrolled hypertension may result in drug discontinuation.[31]

* Altered hemostasis
  * Signs and symptoms: thrombosis, embolism, central nervous system (CNS) bleeding, epistaxis, hematemesis, hemoptysis, and bleeding at tumor sites[31]
  * Characteristics: May occur without warning
  * Treatment: Assess patient before and during treatment; monitor hematologic tests.[31]

* Headache
  * Signs, symptoms, and characteristics: may occur without warning
  * Treatment: Treat symptomatically; premedication before infusion may be helpful.[31]

Iressa

❖ Recommended regimen: (investigational in the treatment of colorectal cancer)

  ❖ 250 mg to 500 mg PO daily.[31]

❖ Common toxicities: acne-like rash, nausea, vomiting, bone pain, fatigue, and diarrhea[31]

❖ Acne-like rash

  ❖ Signs and symptoms: rash, folliculitis, and maculopapular lesions on the face or trunk, especially the upper chest and back[31]

  ❖ Characteristics: Common, occurs in about 60% of patients. Usually mild. Reversible when drug is discontinued.[31]

  ❖ Treatment: No recommended treatment, except cosmetic measures, at this time. Patient education is important, especially due to the emotional impact of this visible skin reaction.

❖ Miscellaneous toxicities: Nausea, vomiting, and diarrhea are usually mild and treated with standard measures.[31] See Table 12-1 and 12-2 for common agents.

General Considerations for Nurses Caring for Patients Being Treated for Colorectal Cancer

❖ Overcome barriers to symptom management

❖ Patient assessment must begin before treatment begins and continue throughout therapy.

❖ Therapeutic interventions must be reevaluated frequently for compliance and effectiveness. Interventions may be evidence-based, anecdotal, or creative solutions to a problem. Even "unprovide measures," when implemented for an individual, can reduce distress.

❖ Consider caregiver burden and the patient's struggles with self-care when recommending interventions

❖ Remember clinical experience indicates that toxicities and symptom experiences vary from patient to patient, so take all side effects seriously and treat them promptly.

❖ Provide clear explanations of self-care measures

❖ Be persistent in attempts to control symptoms. It is not a failure to keep trying strategies to manage a symptom until one is found that works.

❖ Cultural diversity and the wishes and goals of the patient must also be considered when planning care.

❖ To improve care, patients request that we:[32]
   ❖ Be accessible
   ❖ Discover a cure
   ❖ Provide support groups
   ❖ Reinforce current education
   ❖ Provide additional coping strategies
   ❖ Increase patient participation in decision making

❖ Remember the patient surviving with cancer is facing a serious, probably life-threatening illness.

Listen, be empathetic, and provide the best physical and psychological care possible, and you will make a difference in the life of a patient.

References

1. Rhodes VA, and Watson PM. "Symptom Distress—The Concept: Past and Present." *Semin Oncol Nurs.* 1987; 3: 242–247.

2. Ozer H, Armitage JO, Bennett CL, *et al.* "2000 Update of Recommendations for the Use of Hematopoietic Colony-Stimulating Factors: Evidence-Based, Clinical Practice Guidelines." *Journal of Clinical Oncology.* 2000; 18(20): 3558–3585.

3. Wickham RS, Rehwaldt M, Kefer C, *et al.* "Taste Changes Experienced by Patients Receiving Chemotherapy." *Oncol Nurs Forum.* 1999; 26(4): 697–706.

4. Lin EM. "Constipation." In Yasko JM, ed. *Nursing Management of Symptoms Associated with Chemotherapy*, 5th ed. West Conshohocken, PA: Meniscus Limited, 2001: 95–108.

5. Berg DT. "Diarrhea." In Yasko JM, ed. *Nursing Management of Symptoms Associated with Chemotherapy*, 5th ed. West Conshohocken, PA: Meniscus Limited, 2001: 109–130.

6. Krebs LU. "Sexuality and Reproductive Issues." In Yasko JM, ed. *Nursing Management of Symptoms Associated with Chemotherapy*, 5th ed. West Conshohocken, PA: Meniscus Limited, 2001: 205–214.

7. Pharmacia Oncology. Camptosar (irinotecan hydrochloride) [package insert]. Peapack, NJ: Pharmacia Oncology, 2002.

8. Tournigand C, Louvet C, Quinaux E, *et al.* FOLFIRI Followed by FOLFOX Versus FOLFOX Followed by FOLFIRI in Metastatic Colorectal Cancer: Final Results

of a Phase III Study." *Proceedings of ASCO.* 2001; 20: 124a, abstract 494.

9. Goel S, Jhawer M, Rajdev L, *et al.* Phase I Clinical Trial of Irinotecan with Oral Capecitabine in Patients with Gastrointestinal and Other Solid Malignancies." *American Journal of Clinical Oncology.* 2002, in press.

10. Eisnenberg SG, and Marshall JL. "Combination Chemotherapy for Colon Cancer Utilizing a Two-weeks-on, One-week-off Schedule of Irinotecan, 5-Fluorouracil, and Leucovorin: Possible Solution to Reduce Toxicity." *Advances in Colon Cancer.* 2001; 5(2): 3–6.

11. Berg DT, and Lilienfeld C. "Therapeutic Options for Treating Advanced Colorectal Cancer." *Clinical Journal of Oncology Nursing.* 2000; 4(5): 209–216.

12. Petit RG, Rothenberg ML, Mitchell EP, *et al.* "Cholinergic Symptoms Following CPT-11 Infusion in the Phase II Multicenter Trial of 250 mg/m^2 Irinotecan Given Every Two Weeks." *Proc Am Soc Clin Oncol.* 1997; 16: 953 (abstr).

13. Pharmacia Oncology. [Data on file]. Peapack, NJ: Pharmacia Oncology, 1999.

14. Tropea JN, Hoey D, Baumgartel W, *et al.* "Amelioration of Irinotecan Induced Delayed Onset Diarrhea with Oral Sugar and Salt Containing Fluids in Patients with Metastatic Colorectal Cancer." *Proc Am Soc Clin Oncol.* 2002; 21: 255b (abstr 2839).

15. Govindarajan R, Maddox AM, Safar AM, *et al.* "The Efficacy of Thalidomide and Irinotecan In Metastatic Colorectal Carcinoma (Phase II Study)." *Proc Am Soc Clin Oncol.* 2002; 20: 102b (abstr 2222).

16. Berg DT. "Systemic Chemotherapy for Colorectal Cancer." In Berg DT. ed. *Contemporary Issues in Colorectal Cancer: A Nursing Perspective.* Boston, MA: Jones and Bartlett Publishers. 2001: 157–190.

17. Roche Laboratories, Inc. Xeloda (capecitabine) tablets [product insert]. Nutley, NJ: Roche Laboratories, Inc. Available at www.xeloda.com. Accessed July 20, 2002.

18. Timmerman D. "Capecitabine (Xeloda)." *Clin J Oncol Nurs.* 2001; 5(1): 36–37.

19. Lauman MK, and Mortimer J. "Effect of Pyridoxine on the Incidence of Palmar Plantar Erythroderma in Patients Receiving Capecitabine." *Proc Am Soc Clin Oncol.* 2001; 20: 392a (abstr 1565).

20. Lin EH, Morris J, Chau NK, *et al.* "Celecoxib Attenuated Capecitabine Induced Hand-and-Foot Syndrome and Diarrhea and Improved Time to Tumor Progression in Metastatic Colorectal Cancer." *Proc Am Soc Clin Oncol.* 2002; 21: 138b (abstr 2364).

21. De Gramont A, Figer A, Seymour M, *et al.* "Leucovorin and Fluorouracil with or Without Oxaliplatin as First-line Treatment in Advanced Colorectal Cancer." *Journal of Clinical Oncology.* 2000; 18(16); 2938–2947.

22. FDA Eloxatin™ (oxaliplatin for injection). Available at www.fda.gov/cder/drug/infopage/eloxatin. Accessed August 15, 2002.

23. Gamelin E, Gamelin L, Delva R, *et al.* "Prevention of Oxaliplatin Peripheral Sensory Neuropathy by CA+ Gluconate/Mg+ Chloride Infusions: A Retrospective Study." *Proc Am Soc Clin Oncol.* 2002; 21: 157a (abstr 624).

24. Wilkes GM. "New Therapeutic Options in Colon Cancer: Focus on Oxaliplatin." *Clinical Journal of Oncology Nursing.* 2002; 6(3): 131–137.

25. Mariani G, Garrone O, Granetto C, *et al.* "Oxaliplatin Induced Neuropathy: Could Gabapentin Be the Answer?" *Proc Am Soc Clin Oncol.* 2000; 19: 609a (abstr 2397).

26. Dold F, Hoey D, Carberry M, *et al.* "Hypersensitivity in Patients with Metastatic Colorectal Carcinoma

Undergoing Chemotherapy with Oxaliplatin." *Proc Am Soc Clin Oncol.* 2002; 21: 370a (abstr 1478).

27. Saltz L, Meropol NJ, Loehrer PJ, *et al.* "Single Agent IMC-C225 Has Activity in CPT-11-Refractory Colorectal Cancer That Expresses the Epidermal Growth Factor Receptor." *Proc Am Soc Clin Oncol.* 2002; 21: 127a (abstr 2364).

28. Hollywood E. "Clinical Issues in the Administration of an Anti-epidermal Growth Factor Receptor Monoclonal Antibody, IMC-C225." *Seminars in Oncology Nursing.* 2002; 18(2 suppl 2): 30–35.

29. Nirenberg A. "Thalidomide: When Everything Old Is New Again." *Clin J Oncol Nurs.* 2001: 5(1): 15–18.

30. Whitley P, Nirenberg A, Mayorga J, *et al. Thalidomide Nursing Roundtable Report.* Stamford, CT: PharmaCom Group Inc., 2000.

31. CancersourceRN.com. "2002 Oncology Nursing Drug Database." Available at http://www.cancersourcern.com/drugdb/index.cfm. Accessed June 28, 2002.

32. Ferrell B, Grant M, Schmidt GM, *et al.* "The Meaning of Quality of Life for Bone Marrow Transplant Survivors. Part 2: Improving Quality of Life for Bone Marrow Transplant Survivors." *Cancer Nurs.* 1992; 15(4): 247–253.

33. Sanofi~Synthelabo. [Data on file]. New York, NY: Author, 1998.

34. Rosenoff S. "CID Symptom Resolution with Long-Acting Octreotide Depot." *Proc Am Soc Clin Oncol.* 2002; 21: 387a (abstr 1545).

13

Quality of Life Issues for Individuals with Colorectal Cancer

Introduction

Colorectal carcinoma (CRC) is a common and significant health problem for individuals in the United States. It is the only major disease in the United States that almost equally affects men and women. Improvements in treatment have been realized recently, yet an objective tumor response may not translate into freedom from distress and suffering, alterations in quality of life (QOL). A lot is known about survival rates and treatment complications, but little is known about how individuals with CRC adapt to the cancer experience. Interest in QOL is an emerging phenomenon as people are living longer with this disease.

Clinical Implications of Treatment and QOL

❖ Research supports that cancer and its treatment affect the QOL of individuals with CRC.[1]

❖ Treatment response, toxicity of treatment, and duration of freedom from active disease will impact an individual's QOL for the remainder of their life span.

❖ Several components influence patient satisfaction with their treatment:[2]

  ❖ Symptom relief
  ❖ Accessibility to care
  ❖ Treatment environment
  ❖ Interpersonal aspects of care
  ❖ Patient education
  ❖ Mode of chemotherapy administration

  1. Intravenous administration is preferred over continuous pump infusion. Oral administration is most preferred if it is equally efficacious.

❖ The most frequently reported issues for caregivers are:[3]

  ❖ Information about what to do for the patient at home
  ❖ Information about when to expect symptoms to occur
  ❖ Information about who can help them with problems and concerns

❖ The available data speaks more to the physical and psychological aspects of CRC than the social and spiritual dimensions.

   ❖ During treatment, there are many potential physical symptoms; e.g., pain, nausea, fatigue, diarrhea; emotional symptoms, e.g., poor body image, fear, anxiety, and depression; as well as other demands of the illness, e.g., financial, job security, and changes in roles and relationships.[4]

   ❖ At some point in their cancer experience, most patients face issues of uncertainty about the future (and present), ways to reestablish themselves with their family and friends, employability and/or reentry into the workplace, financial problems, life and health insurance difficulties, and for a few, the development of second cancers.

Considerations with Specific Treatment Modalities

❖ Surgery

   ❖ Pretreatment QOL scores predict surgical complications; patients with lower QOL suffered more frequent surgical complications.[5]

   ❖ Surgery can cause short-term pain and tenderness in the area of the operation, along with temporary constipation or diarrhea.

   ❖ As a result of sphincter-sparing procedures, individuals may suffer from physical impairments of bowel and genitourinary function.[6]

❖ Abdominal perineal resection (APR) is associated with a better QOL in patients with rectal cancer compared to anterior resection. Patients experience less fatigue, gastrointestinal symptoms, insomnia, constipation, and diarrhea and report feeling better overall. Body image problems are more common with the APR procedure.[7] Though considered to be a kinder procedure because the sphincter is spared, patients who underwent an anterior resection reported deterioration in their QOL.

❖ Extensive rectal resection may cause damage to the sympathetic or the pelvic parasympathetic nerves and, thus, cause bladder and sexual dysfunction.[8] In addition, individuals who have damage to the internal and external sphincters tend to have a lower QOL.[9]

❖ Laparoscopy procedures are also considered to be kinder procedures, but a recent report suggests that is true only in the short term. Within the first 2 weeks after surgery, those undergoing the laparoscopy procedure stayed in the hospital for a shorter period and required less pain medication as compared to traditional colectomy. However, over the 2 months after the procedures, there was no difference in QOL.[10]

❖ The need for a colostomy as a result of rectal

cancer surgery is associated with a negative impact on QOL. As it turns out, individuals treated at a hospital with a high rectal surgery volume or associated with higher socioeconomic status were less likely to have a permanent colostomy. The reasons behind these findings need to be elucidated.[11]

❖ Research supports the improvement of QOL at approximately 3 months after surgery, when a statistically significant improvement in emotional functioning was reported.[12]

❖ Radiation therapy

❖ During radiotherapy, fatigue, pain, and drowsiness are experienced and result in a deterioration in functioning, e.g., general activities and work. This information may influence symptom management strategies during radiation therapy.[13]

❖ Multimodality therapy is common for many patients with rectal cancer. The addition of chemotherapy to radiation therapy produces more gastrointestinal toxicities and negatively impacts QOL, i.e., generally feeling ill, reduces compliance with treatment, and reduces daily activities. Interestingly though, the overall perception of QOL was the same between the multimodality treatment and radiation therapy alone.[14]

❖ Skin changes, fatigue, loss of appetite, nausea, diarrhea, intestinal obstruction, or bleeding through the rectum are all acute effects of radiation therapy which can negatively impact the patient's QOL.[8]

❖ Chemotherapy

  ❖ Standard adjuvant chemotherapy regimens do not necessarily have a significant adverse impact on QOL.[15]

  ❖ Randomized clinical trials have shown that chemotherapy improves survival and QOL in advanced colorectal cancer.

    1. Elderly patients tolerate and benefit from treatment in the adjuvant and metastatic setting without a significant impairment in QOL.[16,17]

    2. Chemotherapy can improve survival and provide patients with favorable QOL outcomes.[4]

      a. In one trial, the impact of chemotherapy over best supportive care in terms of QOL was very significant and changed the standard treatment paradigm to early chemotherapy rather than watch and wait.[18]

      b. After three cycles of chemotherapy (usual timeframe for documentation of tumor response), emotional and social functioning seem to improve, while scores representative of treatment-induced toxicity worsen.[19]

❖ Baseline QOL and performance status, as well as other measures of the extent of disease are predictive of survival. Individuals with better QOL scores, performance status, and lesser amounts of disease have a higher survival rate.[20]

❖ Women being treated with 5-FU based chemotherapy are 13% more likely to experience severe toxicity, i.e., stomatitis, leukopenia, alopecia, and diarrhea compared with men.[21] Response rates and survival were the same. The oncologist and patient should consider this information when making treatment decisions.

❖ Out-patient administration of infusional chemotherapy appears to improve quality of life and is very acceptable to patients, as compared to inpatient administration, which is expensive and disruptive to their lifestyle.[22]

❖ Patients receiving treatment at home rather than in an outpatient clinic were significantly more satisfied with their care. There were no differences in toxicity, use of healthcare resources, or QOL, and the patients being treated at home reported better communication with their nurses.[23]

Recent Research into the Effects of Some Specific Chemotherapy Regimens on QOL

❖ In the adjuvant setting, 12 weeks of continuous infusion 5-FU ($300 \ mg/m^2/day$) was at least equal to 6 months of 5-FU (425 mg/m^2 IV) and leucovorin [LV] (20 mg/m^2) day 1–5 once a month while producing less toxicity and less impact on QOL.[24]

❖ Continuing infusional 5-FU chemotherapy for metastatic CRC indefinitely until disease progression shows no benefit but does negatively impact QOL and results in increased toxicity. The authors recommended stopping chemotherapy after 12 weeks.[25]

❖ Infusional 5-FU based therapies, either Lokich (continuous infusion daily) or deGramont (2 day infusion every 2 weeks), are equally effective in terms of response and survival. Both regimens relieved pain, anxiety, and improved physical and social functioning in the QOL analysis. Neither improved fatigue or depression. The Lokich regimen had a higher incidence of hand and foot syndrome and central line complications.[26,27]

❖ The addition of irinotecan to bolus 5-FU and LV as first-line treatment sustains overall QOL while improving efficacy and survival as compared with 5-FU and LV given days 1–5 once a month.[28] The results of this trial led to a change in the standard of care for patients with metastatic disease.[29]

❖ Patients treated with infusional 5-FU and LV had a slightly better QOL score than patients treated with infusional 5-FU, LV, plus oxaliplatin. Efficacy was better when oxaliplatin was added to 5-FU and LV.[30]

❖ A regimen of infusional 5-FU, LV, and irinotecan improves QOL in terms of role, social, and emotional functioning, whereas the use of infusional 5-FU, LV, and oxaliplatin or irinotecan plus oxaliplatin did not change QOL. These three treatments are considered efficacious with manageable toxicity profiles in patients whose disease progressed on 5-FU based treatment.[31]

❖ QOL and efficacy are not different when irinotecan is given weekly for 4 out of 6 weeks or once every 3 weeks as second-line therapy. The once every 3 weeks regimen has significantly less severe diarrhea, but a slightly higher rate of neutropenia. Early cholinergic symptoms also occur more often on the once every 3 weeks schedule.[32]

❖ Patients report oral chemotherapy would provide them with several benefits important to their QOL: freedom, autonomy, decreased burden, improvement in physical and emotional well-being, and that they would "feel less different from the general population."[2]

Considerations After Treatment Ends

❖ Goal: restoration of optimal physical, emotional, social, and sexual function

❖ If the treatment is a limited endoscopic procedure, the individual may not think much about their situation. If the treatment is an extensive surgery or a multimodality regimen, the impact may be more significant.

❖ Surveillance

  ❖ After the diagnosis it is very important to identify additional tumors at the earliest stage possible, but it is also a cause for anxiety.

    1. The American Society of Clinical Oncology medical monitoring recommendations involve a physical examination every 3–6 months for 3 years, then yearly; colonoscopy within the first year after diagnosis and then every 3–5 years based on the results; carcinembryonic antigen (CEA) every 2–3 months for 2 years, and then as directed by the physician. For individuals with rectal cancer who did not have pelvic radiation therapy, a proctosigmoidoscopy is recommended every 6–12 months.[33]

    2. The act of medical monitoring is a frequent reminder of the cancer diagnosis. This, the fear of bad news, and the possibility of false-positive and false-negative test results can be anxiety provoking.

❖ Regression of Treatment Side Effects

  ❖ Side effects often resolve within weeks after treatment discontinuation, but sometimes they may take months even years to regress. Unfortunately, there are some adverse events that may be permanent.

  ❖ Common acute treatment related complications: diarrhea, nausea, vomiting, fatigue, and hair loss. These are discussed in Chapter 12.

- ❖ Common late complications: adhesions, urinary or fecal incontinence, weakened abdominal muscles post op, fistulae, hernia, sexual dysfunction, and cardiac injury
- ❖ Most individuals with CRC will have an increase in QOL several years after diagnosis (usual by approximately 3 years); however, they may continue to suffer in several areas, particularly pain, ambulation, and social well-being.[34]

❖ Coping with CRC

- ❖ Psychological well-being is often compromised by high levels of generalized distress and negative body image, which is more frequent in women and young adults.[1]
- ❖ Having an ostomy has a negative psychological affect, specifically in terms of body image and sexuality. Men may have erectile dysfunction and ejaculatory difficulties, while women may have dyspareunia.[35]
- ❖ The end of therapy may be a mixed blessing; the patient is glad that therapy is completed, but fearful of having less contact with the healthcare provider without the frequent treatment visits. It is important to help the patient bridge this change in their care.
- ❖ The patient must move on with their normal activities, but for some individuals this is not easy.
- ❖ The fear of recurrence can be overwhelming. Honest discussions about the likelihood of

recurrence can help put this fear into perspective.

❖ Financial issues can put a significant strain on the patient and family. Employability, health-care insurability, and life insurance coverage are all very real issues. Completing applications for disability or future disability in a timely fashion is especially important.

Living with a Stoma

❖ Directions for Changing the Ostomy Bag and Flange, Table 13-1

❖ Activities of Daily Living[36]

❖ Sexual Activity

1. Activity may resume as soon as the patient no longer has abdominal discomfort.
2. In a recent study, only 10% of women but 53.8% of men noted they were unsatisfied with their current sexual activity.[37]
3. Body image changes, for both the patient and partner, may interfere. The partner may also fear hurting the patient. Open communication is important.
4. Avoid gas producing foods, such as those in the broccoli and cabbage family.
5. Empty bag just before activity to prevent likelihood of accident. Note, some patients do not need to wear a bag except for times predictable for bowel movements.

TABLE 13-1
Directions for Changing the Ostomy Bag and Flange

1. Remove the soiled bag and flange.

2. Wash the area around the stoma with mild soap and water. Do not use a soap with a lotion or cream base, as it will prevent the new product from adhering to the skin.

3. Allow the area to dry.

4. Apply skin protector or barrier film. This usually comes as an individually packaged 1-inch pad or in a lollipop form. This protects peristomal skin from erosion from the adhesive barrier and feces.

5. Allow the area to dry.

6. Cut the flange. This is the backing part of the bag that will adhere to the skin. It should be cut one-fourth of an inch larger than the stoma to prevent irritation to the stoma or leakage under the flange. Remove the paper backing from the flange.

7. Apply stoma adhesive paste, if needed. This product comes in a tube and should be applied to the flange adhesive side about one-fourth of an inch in from the edge. Apply like toothpaste and let dry.

8. When the stoma adhesive paste and the skin are totally dry, carefully apply the flange to the skin, making sure the opening is not covering any portion of the stoma.

9. If using the two-piece system, attach the bag and clamp the lower end of the bag.

10. If teaching patients, ask for a return demonstration of steps 1 through 9, as well as having them practice unclamping and clamping the bag as if they were emptying the bag. The bag should be emptied whenever it is half full, to prevent bag explosion. After emptying the bag, wipe the open end with toilet tissue and then reclamp the bag.

Source: Waldman AR, and Crane AE. "Surgical Aspects of Colon Cancer." In Berg DT, ed. *Contemporary Issues in Colorectal Cancer: A Nursing Perspective.* Boston, MA: Jones and Bartlett Publishers. 2001: 105–134.

6. Products are available that will cover the pouch increasing the comfort with intimacy.
7. It is important that patients discuss any problems or concerns with their physician and/or nurse.

❖ Hygiene: Bathing and showering may be done either with or without the pouch in place.[36]
❖ Diet: Usually all foods eaten prior to surgery can be enjoyed afterwards.
❖ Irrigation of the stoma is important to some patients and should be discussed with the physician and/or enterstomal therapy nurse.
❖ Ostomy supplies can be purchased through most drug stores, medical supply stores, or ordered through the mail. It is important to always make sure there are enough supplies still on hand when purchasing additional supplies in case the order is delayed.
❖ Work and social activities: There are commonly no restrictions on participation in social activities or work. Patients should avoid very heavy lifting, however.
❖ Sport Activities: Ostomy bags often have hooks and a belt which can be inserted into the hooks and worn around the waist for extra security. With the assistance of such ostomy bags, ostomates can participate in almost all types of sports, with the exception of heavy body contact sports.[36]

Selected Symptoms Resulting from Progressive Disease

❖ The patient with advanced or progressive disease needs assistance in achieving freedom from pain, both physical and psychological. Relief of physical pain is often easier to achieve. Fear, anxiety, depression, anger, and loneliness may be more challenging to alleviate. Often the patient and family seek answers about how much time is left, what will it be like in the end; however, no one can truly predict the tumor growth rate and the resulting duration of life. Palliative care to support the patient physically as well as emotionally is very important to maintain QOL for as long as possible.

❖ Table 13-2 offers nursing interventions for select symptoms.

Future Directions

❖ There is an increasing need to assess the impact of the disease and its treatment in patients' and families' QOL

❖ QOL data gained from a clinical trial can help inform patients and healthcare providers about common concerns and reactions to specific treatments. This information can be used to help

TABLE 13-2
Nursing Interventions for Select Symptoms.

Symptom	Nursing Interventions
Ascites	1. Complete a baseline abdominal examination, noting girth and reevaluate regularly.
	2. Instruct the patient to report any changes in breathing; early satiety; abdominal bloating; new, unexplained weight gain; fit of clothes; difficulty walking; and edema.
	3. Monitor and maintain fluid and electrolyte balance; minimize sodium and fluid intake.
	4. Assess the patient for peripheral edema; utilize compression stockings and keep the patient's feet and legs elevated; avoid restrictive clothing.
	5. Administer therapy to treat the underlying disease.
	6. Assist with intermittent paracenteses and monitor for complications.
	7. Initiate pain management strategies, as appropriate.
Bowel obstruction	1. Assess the patient for signs and symptoms of bowel obstruction: nausea, sporadic vomiting, abdominal pain, worsening constipation, and lack of bowel sounds.
	2. Explain to the patient with suspected obstruction about the cause and the diagnostic work-up.
	3. Initiate antiemetics, stool softeners, and a soft or liquid diet for early bowel obstruction.

(continued)

TABLE 13-2
Nursing Interventions for Select Symptoms (continued).

Symptom	Nursing Interventions
Bowel obstruction (continued)	4. Intravenous fluids, antiemetics, electrolyte replacement, and nasogastric suctioning are recommended for severe obstruction and vomiting.
	5. Teach the patient about the rationale of nasogastric suctioning and parental fluids.
	6. Assess the patient for complications of bowel obstruction, dehydration, peritonitis, bowel perforation, hypotension, hypovolemia, or septic shock.
	7. If appropriate, prepare the patient for surgery (i.e., colectomy, colostomy, gastrointestinal bypass, and gastric or intestinal tube placement).
	8. If inoperable, a gastrostomy tube or a percutaneous endoscopic gastrostomy tube may be appropriate.[30]
Emotion distress, e.g., fear and anxiety	1. Establish a trusting relationship with the patient.
	2. Assess the patient's levels of fear, anxiety, and psychosocial worries by asking general therapeutic questions, such as, "What are your concerns about your illness?"
	3. Listen to and acknowledge the patient's and family's feelings, struggles, and concerns.
	4. Clarify misconceptions about their disease status and develop realistic goals.

(continued)

TABLE 13-2
Nursing Interventions for Select Symptoms (continued).

Symptom	Nursing Interventions
Emotion distress, e.g., fear and anxiety (continued)	5. Assure the patient that he or she will receive palliative therapies, as appropriate.
	6. Provide emotional support, consulting with a social worker and other healthcare providers as needed.
	7. Assist the patient in managing emotional stress and maintaining equilibrium.
	8. Encourage the patient to get his or her affairs "in order" legally.
	9. Initiate a referral for a visiting nurse, home health aide, and hospice, as appropriate.
Fatigue	1. Determine the possible etiology of fatigue.
	2. Develop a trusting relationship to facilitate open discussion.
	3. Prescribe treatment based on underlying etiology and evaluate its effectiveness.
	4. Teach the patient to rest, as needed, throughout the day, yet maintain normal bedtime patterns and rituals.
	5. Educate the patient that fatigue may linger after treatment is completed.
	6. Encourage an individualized exercise program.
	7. Instruct the patient to eat nutritionally balanced foods especially those high in iron, such as liver, eggs, carrots, and raisins.

(continued)

TABLE 13-2
Nursing Interventions for Select Symptoms (continued).

Symptom	Nursing Interventions
Fatigue (continued)	8. Advise the patient to do the following: ◆ Prioritize activities throughout day, avoiding overexertion. ◆ Schedule the most important activities at times of maximal energy levels. ◆ Delegate activities and responsibilities to family members and friends. ◆ Create strategies to overcome "energy drainers": for example, eliminate stair climbing; get assistance, as needed, with personal hygiene and dressing; and allow friends and family members to prepare meals and do laundry.[38] 9. Initiate a referral for a visiting nurse and home health aide, as appropriate.
Pain	1. Using a consistent assessment tool, assess the patient's pain: onset, location, severity, intensity, duration, and any associated symptoms. 2. Evaluate conditions or interventions that alleviate the discomfort. 3. Initiate appropriate interventions based on assessment. 4. Administer analgesics and routine and rescue medications on schedule, as prescribed. Morphine sulfate is the drug of choice for severe pain.[39] 5. Educate the patient about the common side effects of most pain regimens and self-care measures to treat them.

(continued)

TABLE 13-2
Nursing Interventions for Select Symptoms (continued).

Symptom	Nursing Interventions
Pain (continued)	6. Utilize nonpharmacologic methods to reduce pain: heat and cold, rest, music therapy, humor therapy, hypnosis, acupuncture, progressive muscle relaxation, guided imagery, and distraction.
	7. Evaluate the effectiveness of the interventions and alter the plan of care, as needed.
Pruritus	1. Monitor the patient's bilirubin levels and report abnormalities to the physician.
	2. Differentiate between pruritus from an accumulation of bile salts and other etiologies of skin reactions.
	3. Administer therapy, as ordered, to treat the underlying malignancy.
	4. Encourage the patient to increase fluid intake and to avoid alcohol and smoking.
	5. Initiate symptomatic measures to control or prevent the patient's itching.
	◆ Apply topical anesthetic or corticosteroid preparations, as prescribed.
	◆ Cholestyramine may relieve pruritus from hepatic abnormalities.
	6. Evaluate the effectiveness of the interventions.

(continued)

TABLE 13-2
Nursing Interventions for Select Symptoms (continued).

Symptom	Nursing Interventions
Thrombophlebitis and pulmonary embolism	1. Determine the patient's risk of developing DVT.[33] Risk increased with: ◆ Diagnosis of colon or rectal cancer ◆ Sedentary lifestyle ◆ History of abnormalities in clotting or previous DVT ◆ Injury or trauma to vasculature or extremity ◆ Treatment used to treat malignancy (e.g., abdominal surgery, chemotherapy) ◆ History of cigarette smoking 2. Assess the patient for chest pain and/or shortness of breath. 3. Assess the patient's calf for signs of thrombosis. 4. Instruct the patient to wear antiembolism stockings when in bed and to perform leg exercises. 5. Encourage regular exercise and ambulation to prevent stasis. 6. Educate the patient about the radiographic work-up if DVT is suspected. 7. Administer anticoagulant therapy, as prescribed, paying particular attention to dosing at consistent times, while monitoring coagulation parameters. 8. Educate the patient about self-injection of anticoagulant therapy while at home.

(continued)

TABLE 13-2
Nursing Interventions for Select Symptoms (continued).

Symptom	Nursing Interventions
Thrombophlebitis and pulmonary embolism (continued)	9. Assess the patient's compliance with prescribed interventions.
Ureteral obstruction	1. Assess the patient's urinary output and serum creatinine.
	2. If ureteral obstruction is suspected, educate the patient about the underlying cause and the diagnostic work-up.
	3. Educate the patient about urinary stents or nephrostomy tubes, if inserted.
	◆ Cleanse and dress the site according to hospital policy.
	◆ Tape tubes securely in place.
	◆ Assess the site for signs of infection, reduced urinary output, blockage, or bleeding. Report any changes to the physician or nurse.
	◆ Flush tubes, as ordered, according to hospital policy.
	4. Monitor BUN, creatinine, and electrolytes. Notify the physician of abnormalities.

Source: Hogan CM, and Berg DT. "Advanced Disease: Symptom Management Strategies." In Berg DT, ed. *Contemporary Issues in Colorectal Cancer: A Nursing Perspective.* Boston, MA: Jones and Bartlett Publishers, 2001: 241–254.

newly diagnosed individuals to make medical decisions between treatment options.

The Role for Nursing

❖ Goals: Provide holistic and supportive care to patients and families throughout the trajectory of their illness.

   ❖ Clinical experience indicates that the diagnosis of colorectal cancer affects the physical, psychological, social, and spiritual well-being of patients.

   ❖ Nurse must adapt clinical practice and patient education by what is currently known regarding the QOL of individuals living with colorectal cancer.

   ❖ Table 13-3 displays some recommendations for oncology nurses to improve the QOL for individuals with colorectal cancer.

   ❖ More needs to be learned about how patients with CRC adapt during their cancer experience. What is known is that all individuals with colorectal cancer may suffer physical effects while undergoing treatment. These side effects or symptoms ultimately can negatively affect QOL. With clinical expertise and emotional support, nurses can have a positive impact in the life of the patient and family.

TABLE 13-3
Recommendations to Improve Quality of Life for Individuals with
Colorectal Cancer

Be present and list to patient's concerns.

Assess the patient's view of QOL (physical, psychological,
social, and spiritual).

Help patients and families identify what makes their QOL
better or worse.

Encourage patients to participate in activities that improve
QOL.

Be respectful and honest.

Serve as an advocate.

Ask about body image and sexuality issues.

Ask about and help with any concerns if the patient has an
ostomy.

Provide education and information (concentrate on concrete
objective information).

Help the patient derive hope.

Help the patient to accomplish their goals.

Assist with religious and/or spiritual issues.

Care for the family as well as the patient.

Encourage support from the patient's family and friends.

Provide support groups for patients and families.

Be aware of and manage symptoms and potential long-term
effects of treatment and the impact on QOL.

Provide appropriate skin care if the individual is receiving
radiation therapy.

Source: King CR. "Quality of Life Issues for Individuals with Colorectal
Cancer." In Berg DT, ed. *Contemporary Issues in Colorectal Cancer: A Nursing
Perspective.* Boston, MA: Jones and Bartlett Publishers, 2001: 223–236.
Reprinted with permission.

References

1. Sprangers MAG. "Quality of Life Assessment in Colorectal Cancer Patients: Evaluation of Cancer Therapies." *Semin Oncol.* 1999; 26(3): 691–696.

2. Tredeau E, Seignobos E, Evans C, *et. al.* "Factors That Influence Patient Satisfaction in Colorectal Cancer Patients." *Proceedings ASCO.* 2002; 21: 142b (abstract 2380).

3. Osenenko P, Hwang SS, Chang VT, *et al.* "Caregiver's Unmet Needs and Its Correlation with Caregiver Burden and Satisfaction in Symptomatic Advanced Cancer Patients." *Proceedings ASCO.* 2002; 21: 255b (abstract 2837).

4. King CR. "Quality of Life Issues for Individuals with Colorectal Cancer." In Berg DT. ed. *Contemporary Issues in Colorectal Cancer: A Nursing Perspective.* Boston, MA: Jones and Bartlett Publishers, 2001: 223–236.

5. Anthony T, Leitch AM, Hynan L, *et al.* "Pretreatment Health-Related Quality of Life Is Associated with Surgical Complications in Patients with Colorectal Cancer." *Proceedings ASCO.* 2002; 21: 250a (abstract 997).

6. Sprangers MAG, Taal BG, Aaronson NK, *et al.* "Quality of Life in Colorectal Cancer. Stoma vs Nonstoma Patients." *Dis Colon Rectum.* 1995; 38: 361–369.

7. Reuters News. "Extensive Resection Does not Yield Worse Quality of Life for Rectal Cancer Patients." February 22, 2001. Available at http://www.cancer-source.com/NewsFeatures/News/detail.cfm?DiseaseID=3&Contentid=21871. Accessed July 6, 2002.

8. DeCrosse JJ, and Cennerazzo WJ. "Quality of Life Management of Patients with Colorectal Cancer." *CA Cancer J Clin.* 1997; 47: 198–206.

9. Shibata D, Guillem JG, Lanouette BS, *et al*. "Functional and Quality of Life Outcomes in Patients with Rectal Cancer After Combined Modality Therapy, Intraoperative Radiation Therapy, and Sphincter Preservation." *Dis Colon Rectum*. 2000; 43(6): 752–758.

10. Reuters News. "No Life-quality Benefit with Colon Surgery Method." January 16, 2002. Available at http://www.cancersource.com/NewsFeatures/News/detail.cfm?DiseaseID=3&Contentid=24330. Accessed July 6, 2002.

11. Hodgson DC, Zhang W, Fuchs CS, *et al*. "The Effect of Hospital Volume and Socioeconomic Status on Colostomy Rates for Rectal Cancer." *Proceedings ASCO*. 2001; 20: 238a (abstract 951).

12. Whyness DK, and Neilson AR. "Symptoms Before and After Surgery for Colorectal Cancer." *Qual Life Res*. 1997; 6: 61–66.

13. Reyes-Gibby C, Cleeland CS, Wang X, *et al*. "Symptom Patterns and Their Impact on the Quality of Life Among Patients Receiving Radiotherapy." *Proceedings ASCO*. 2001; 20: 314b (abstract 3007).

14. Caffo O, Amichetti M, Romano M, *et al*. "Evaluation of Quality of Life During Adjuvant Chemotherapy Plus Concurrent Radiotherapy for Resected Rectal Cancer: Results from a Prospective Pilot Study." *Proceedings ASCO*. 2000; 19: 287a (abstract 1124).

15. Gray R, Watson M, McConkey C, *et al*. "Adjuvant Chemotherapy for Colorectal Cancer Has only Minor Impact on Patient Reported Quality of Life: A Study of 785 Patients Randomized in the UKCCCRR QUASAR Trial." *Proceedings ASCO*. 2001; 20: 407a (abstract 1623).

16. Watters JM, Cripps MC, O'Rourke K, *et al*. "Functional Status Is Well Maintained in Older Patients During

Adjuvant Therapy for Colorectal Cancer." *Proceedings ASCO.* 2002; 21: 365a (abstract 1457).

17. Berretta M, Buonadonna A, Rupolo M, *et al.* "Comparison Between Elderly and Non-Elderly Patients, of Efficacy and Tolerability of FOLFOX2 Schedule in Advanced Colorectal Cancer." *Proceedings ASCO.* 2001; 20: 111b (abstract 2195).

18. Cunningham D. "Setting a New Standard-Irinotecan (Campto) in the Second-Line Therapy of Colorectal Cancer: Final Results of Two Phase II Studies and Implications for Clinical Practice." *Semin Oncol.* 1999; 26(1): 1–5 (suppl 5).

19. Kim JS, Kim BS, Choi IK, *et al.* "Changes of Quality of Life and Factors Affecting Quality of Life During Chemotherapy in Cancer Patients." *Proceedings ASCO.* 1999; 18: 599a (abstract 2314).

20. Allen M, Maisey N, Norman A, *et al.* "Baseline Quality of Life Predicts Survival in Patients with Advanced Colorectal Cancer." *Proceedings ASCO.* 2001; 20: 207b (abstract 2580).

21. Reuters News. "Toxicity of 5-FU-Based Chemotherapy More Severe in Women than Men." April 5, 2002. Available at http://www.cancersource.com/ NewsFeatures/News/detail.cfm?Diseaseid=3&Contentid =24805. Accessed July 6, 2002.

22. Rowe MJ, and James RD. "Acceptability of Intermittent Infusion Chemotherapy for Metastatic Colorectal Cancer as an Out-Patient Procedure: A Pilot Study." *Proceedings ASCO.* 1999; 18: 605a (abstract 22338).

23. Reuters News. "At-home Administration of Chemotherapy Improves Patient Satisfaction." April 10, 2001. Available at http://www.cancersource.com/ NewsFeatures/News/detail.cfm?DiseaseID=3&Contentid =22229. Accessed July 6, 2002.

24. Saini A, Cunningham D, Norman AR, *et al.* "Multicentre Randomized Trial of Protracted Venous Infusion 5-FU Compared to 5-FU/Folinic Acid as Adjuvant Therapy for Colorectal Cancer." *Proceedings ASCO.* 2000; 19: 240a (abstract 928).

25. Maughan TS, James RD, Kerr DJ, *et al.* "Continuous vs Intermittent Chemotherapy for Advanced Colorectal Cancer: Preliminary Results of the MRC Cr06b Randomised Trial." *Proceedings ASCO.* 2001; 20: 125a (abstract 498).

26. Maughan TS, James RD, Kerr DJ, *et al.* "Comparison of Survival, Palliation, and Quality of Life with Three Chemotherapy Regimens in Metastatic Colorectal Cancer: A Multicentre Randomised Trial." *The Lancet.* 2002; 359)9317): 1555–1563.

27. Stephens RJ, Hopwood P, Johnston C, *et al.* "The Value of Quality of Life Outcomes in Comparing 3 Chemotherapy Regimens (De Gramont, Lokich, and Ralititrexed) in a Multicentre Randomised Trial of Metastatic Colorectal Cancer." *Proceedings ASCO.* 1999; 18: 575a (abstract 2220).

28. Locker PK, Miller LL, Pirotta N, *et al.* "Weekly Irinotecan Combined with 5-Fluorouracil and Leucovorin in Patients with Untreated Metastatic Colorectal Cancer: Impact on Quality of Life." *Proceedings ASCO.* 2000; 19: 620a (abstract 2443).

29. Saltz LB, Cox JV, Blanke C, *et al.* "Irinotecan Plus Fluorouracil and Leucovorin for Metastatic Colorectal Cancer." *N Engl J Med.* 2000; 343(13): 905–914.

30. Seymour MT, Tabah-Fisch I, Homerin M, *et al.* "Quality of Life in Advanced Colorectal Cancer: A Comparison of Quality of Life During Bolus Plus Infusion 5-FU/Leucovorin with or Without Oxaliplatin." *Proceedings ASCO.* 1999; 18: 234a (abstract 901).

31. Rougier P, Lepille D, Douillard JY, *et al.* "Final Results of a Randomised Phase II Study of Three Combinations: CPT-11 + LV5FU2, LOHP + LV5FU2, and CPT-11 + LOHP in 5-FU Resistant Advanced Colorectal Cancer." *Proceedings ASCO.* 2001; 20: 142a (abstract 566).

32. Fuchs, CS, Hecht JR, Moore MR, *et al.* "Phase III Comparison of Two CPT-11 Dosing Regimens (Weekly × 4 Every-6-weeks vs Every-3-weeks) in Second-Line Metastatic Colorectal Cancer Therapy." *Proceedings ASCO.* 2002; 21: 129a (abstract 514).

33. American Society of Clinical Oncology. *A Patient's Guide: Follow up Care for Colorectal Cancer.* Alexandria, VA: ASCO, 2001.

34. Ramsey SD, Andersen MR, Etzioni R, *et al.* "Quality of Life in Survivors of Colorectal Carcinoma." *Cancer.* 2000; 88(6): 1303.

35. Sprunk E, and Alteneder RR. "The Impact of an Ostomy on Sexuality." *Clin J Oncol Nurs.* 2000; 4(2): 85–88.

36. United Ostomy Association. "UOA Fact Sheets, Colostomy." February 26, 2002. Available at http://www.uoa.org/ostomyinfo.shtml. Accessed June 30, 2002.

37. Krouse RS, Grube B, Grant M, et al. "Ostomy Related Sexual Dysfunction: An Important Quality of Life Issue." *Proceedings ASCO.* 1999; 18: 599a (abstract 2316).

38. McDaniel RW, and Rhodes VA. "Fatigue." In Yarbro CH, Frogge MH, Goodman M, *et al.*, eds. *Cancer Nursing: Principles and Practice,* 5th ed. Boston, MA: Jones and Bartlett Publishers, 2000: 737–753.

39. Crowley, MJ. "Symptom Management and Supportive Care: Dying and Death." In Itano JK, Taoka KN, eds. *Core Curriculum for Oncology Nursing*, 3rd ed. Philadelphia, PA: W.B. Saunders Company, 1998: 96–114.

Appendix A

*Select Toxicities from the
National Cancer Institute
(NCI) Common Toxicity
Criteria (CTC) Version 2.0*

Side Effect	Grade 0	Grade 1	Grade 2	Grade 3	Grade 4
Neutrophils	Normal	$\geq 1500-<2000/mm^3$	$\geq 1000-<1500/mm^3$	$\geq 500-<1000/mm^3$	$<500/mm^3$
Leukocytes	Normal	<lower limit of normal to $3.0 \times 10^9/L$	≥ 2.0 to $<3.0 \times 10^9/L$	>1.0 to $<2.0 \times 10^9/L$	$<1.0 \times 10^9/L$
Platelets	Normal	<lower limit of normal to $75,000/mm^3$	$\geq 50,000-<75,000/mm^3$	$\geq 10,000-<50,000/mm^3$	$<10,000/mm^3$
Stomatitis	None	Painless ulcers, erythema, or mild soreness	Painful erythema, edema, or ulcers but able to eat	Painful erythema, edema or ulcers, and cannot eat	Requires parenteral or enteral support
Diarrhea without a colostomy	None	Increase of <4 stools/day over pretreatment	Increase of 4-6 stools/day over pretreatment	Increase of >7 stools/day over pretreatment; or need for parenteral support for dehydration	Physiologic consequences requiring intensive care; or hemodynamic collapse

(continued)

Side Effect	Grade 0	Grade 1	Grade 2	Grade 3	Grade 4
Diarrhea with a colostomy	None	Mild increase in loose, watery colostomy output compared with pretreatment	Moderate increase in loose, watery colostomy output compared with pretreatment, but not interfering with normal activity	Severe increase in loose, watery colostomy output compared with pretreatment, interfering with normal activity	Physiologic consequences requiring intensive care; or hemodynamic collapse
Nausea	None	Able to eat	Oral intake significantly reduced	No significant oral intake; IVF required	NA
Vomiting	None	1 episode in 24 hours over baseline	2–5 episodes in 24 hours over baseline	>6 episodes in 24 hours over baseline; or need for IV fluids	Requiring parenteral nutrition; or physiologic consequences requiring intensive care; hemo-dynamic collapse

(continued)

Side Effect	Grade 0	Grade 1	Grade 2	Grade 3	Grade 4
Hand Foot Syndrome	None	Skin changes, erythema, peeling, or dermatitis without pain	Skin changes with pain, but not interfering with daily activities	Skin changes with pain, interfering with daily activities	NA
Allergic reaction/Hyper-sensitivity	None	Transient rash, drug fever <100.4°F	Urticaria, drug fever >100.4°F, and/or asymptomatic bronchospasm	Symptomatic bronchospasm requiring parenteral treatment, with or without urticaria; allergy related edema/angioedema	anaphylaxis
Pigmentation changes	None	Localized changes	Generalized changes	NA	NA
Photosensi-tivity	None	Painless erythema	Painful erythema	Erythema with desquamation	NA
Radiation dermatitis	None	Faint erythema or dry desquamation	Moderate erythema or patchy moist desquamation, mostly confined to skin folds and creases; moderate edema	Confluent moist desquamation ≥1.5 cm diameter and not confined to skin folds and creases; pitting edema	Skin necrosis or ulceration of full thickness dermis; may include bleeding not induced by trauma or abrasion

(continued)

Side Effect	Grade 0	Grade 1	Grade 2	Grade 3	Grade 4
Rash/desquamation	None	Macular or papular eruption or erythema without other symptoms	Macular or papular eruption, erythema with itchiness or other symptoms, localized desquamation, or other lesions covering <50% of the skin	Symptomatic generalized erythroderma or macular, papular, or vesicular eruption or desquamation covering ≥50% of the skin	Generalized exfoliative dermatitis or ulcerative dermatitis
Fatigue	None	Increased fatigue compared with baseline, but not affecting activities of daily living	Moderate, e.g., decrease in performance status (1 level ECOG or 20% Karnofsky) **or** causing some difficulty with activities of daily living	Severe, e.g., decrease in performance status (≥2 level ECOG or 40% Karnofsky) **or** causing some difficulty with activities of daily living	Bedridden, disabling

Appendix B

National Cancer Institute Performance Scale

ECOG		Karnofsky	
Score	Description	Score	Description
0	Fully active; able to carry on all pre-disease activities without restriction	100	Normal, no complaints, no evidence of disease
		90	Able to carry on normal activity; minor signs or symptoms of disease
1	Restricted in physically strenuous activity but ambulatory and able to carry out work of a light or sedentary nature, e.g., light housework, office work	80	Normal activity with effort; some signs or symptoms of disease
		70	Cares for self, unable to carry on normal activity or do active work

(continued)

ECOG		Karnofsky	
Score	Description	Score	Description
2	Ambulatory and capable of self-care, but unable to carry out any work activities; up and about more than 50% of the day	60	Requires occasional assistance, but is able to care for most of own needs
		50	Requires considerable assistance and frequent medical care
3	Capable of only limited self-care, confined to bed or chair more than 50% of the day	40	Disabled, requires special care and assistance
		30	Severely disabled, hospitalization indicated. Death not imminent.
4	Completely disabled. Cannot perform self-care. Totally confined to bed or chair	20	Very sick, hospitalization indicated. Death not imminent.
		10	Moribund, fatal processes progressing rapidly.

Source: National Cancer Institute Cancer Therapy Evaluation Program. Common Toxicity Criteria Document Version 2.0. Published April 30, 1999. Available at http://ctep.cancer.gov/reporting/ctc.html. Accessed July 12, 2002.

Appendix C

Colorectal Cancer Resources for Patients, Families, and Professionals

Internet Resources

There is a tremendous amount of information available on the Internet, but some of it may not be reliable. Each of the sites listed has been reviewed for content, readability, and timely information.

American Cancer Society

Main Web site address: www.cancer.org

Colorectal cancer specific web site address: http://www.cancer.org/eprise/main/docroot/lrn/lrn-0

Provides patient educational materials, support programs, prevention and cancer awareness information, and treatment center referrals

American College of Gastroenterology

Web site address: www.acg.gi.org

Provides information and referrals regarding colorectal cancer and other digestive conditions

American Society of Clinical Oncology

Web site address: www.asco.org

National organization for oncologists; supports cancer research; provides educational programs and materials; supports "People Living with Cancer" Web site: http://www.peoplelivingwithcancer.org/plwc/Home/0,47466,,00.html

American Society of Colon and Rectal Surgeons

Web site address: www.fascrs.org

Patient information available regarding colon and rectal surgery and other gastrointestinal conditions

American Society for Gastrointestinal Endoscopy

Web site address: www.asge.org

Patient information about the use of endoscopy to diagnose and treat gastrointestinal diseases

American Society of Therapeutic Radiation and Oncology

Web site address: www.astro.org

Provides information about cancer and radiation oncology

Association of Community Cancer Centers

Web site address: www.accc-cancer.org/main2001.shtml

Information regarding cancer centers, basic insurance information, treatments, and standards

Cancer Care, Inc.

Web site address: www.cancercare.org

Patient information, counseling, and support groups available; referrals available

Cancer Hope Network

Web site address: www.cancerhopenetwork.org

Trained cancer survivor volunteers provide one-to-one support to cancer patients and their families.

Cancer Research Foundation of America (CRFA)

Web site address: http://www.preventcancer.org/colorectal/aboutcolorectal/aboutcolo.cfm

Provides information about prevention and early detection through research and education

CancerSource.com

Web site address: www.cancersource.com

Comprehensive source of information about cancer, including colorectal cancer; symptom management information, links to clinical trial information, message boards, and live-chats on a variety of topics are available.

Centers for Disease Control

Web site address: www.cdc.gov/cancer/colorctl/index.htm

Information on colorectal cancer prevention and control initiatives; "Screen for Life: National Colorectal Cancer Action Campaign"

Center for Cancer Nutrition

Web site address: www.cancernutrition.com

Certified nutritional specialist provides information about cancer and nutrition

Collaborative Group of the Americas on Inherited Colorectal Cancer (ACG-ICC)

Web site address: www.fascrs.org/ascrs-cancer-reg.html

Provides a listing of hereditary colon cancer registries and information on clinical and chemoprevention clinical trials

Colon Cancer Alliance

Web site address: www.ccalliance.org

Educational information on colorectal cancer topics, support groups, news articles, and links to other cancer organizations

Colorectal Cancer Association of Canada

Web site address: www.ccac-accc.ca

Dedicated to supporting people with colorectal cancer, their families, and caregivers; increase quality of life and cancer awareness

Colorectal Cancer Network

Web site address: www.colorectal-cancer.net

Provides information about treatment options and disease management

Harvard Center for Cancer Prevention

Web site address: www.yourcancerrisk.harvard.edu

Risk assessment for the public

Hereditary Colon Cancer Association

Web site address: www.hereditarycc.org

Provides support and information for patients with an inherited colon cancer disorder and their families

National Cancer Institute

Main Web site address: cancer.gov

Colorectal cancer information Web site address: cancer.gov/cancer_information/cancer_type/colon_and_rectal

Provides information on treatment, prevention, genetics, screening, clinical trials, and links to Cancerlit® literature search.

National Cancer Institute Cancer Information Service (CIS)

Web site address: cis.nci.nih.gov

Provides information on cancer, treatment, and clinical trials

National Cancer Institute Office of Cancer Survivorship

Web site address: <u>dccps.nci.nih.gov/ocs</u>

Defines and coordinates research to improve the quality of life and health of cancer survivors and their families

National Center for Complementary and Alternative Medicine

Web site address: <u>nccam.nih.gov</u>

Provides information on complementary and alternative practices

National Coalition for Cancer Survivorship

Web site address: <u>www.canceradvocacy.org</u>

Advocacy organization for insurance, employment, and legal rights for cancer survivors

National Colon Cancer Research Alliance

Web site address: <u>www.nccra.org</u>

Information on colon cancer and research efforts

National Hospice and Palliative Care Organization

Web site address: www.nhpco.org

Provides public and professional information about hospice and palliative care. Advocates for the terminally ill and their families. Provides referrals to local hospitals, advocacy groups, and professional organizations.

Oncology Nursing Society

Web site address: www.ons.org

National organization promoting excellence in oncology nursing and quality cancer care

*Ph*RMA

Web site address: www.phrma.org

Provides information about prescription medications, including a directory of patient-assistance programs.

The Society of Gastroenterology Nurses and Associates

Web site address: www.sgna.org

Provides information to promote awareness about colorectal cancer.

United Ostomy Association

Web site address: www.uoa.org

Provides information, support, and advocacy for people with ostomies.

The Wellness Community

Web site address: www.wellness-community.org

Provides educational materials, psychosocial support, and social activities to patients and families. The "Frankly Speaking" patient information kit is available from the Wellness Community.

Wound Ostomy and Continence Nurses Society

Web site address: www.wocn.org

National organization of enterostomal therapy nurses; local referrals available

Index